Praise for *Honest Medicine*

In *Honest Medicine*, Julia Schopick writes about four innovative treatments that many cutting-edge integrative doctors have successfully used for years. But never before, to my knowledge, have they been featured together in one book. Any patient who is interested in learning about nontoxic, inexpensive alternatives to costly, side-effective-laden pharmaceuticals should read Julia's book. I predict that *Honest Medicine* will become an instant classic.

—Ronald Hoffman, MD, Author, Founder and Medical Director of
the Hoffman Center in New York, Host of "Health Talk,"
nationally syndicated radio talk show

Patients around the world have a compassionate new advocate and voice in Julia Schopick. Julia is one of those rare people in this world who can go through an agonizingly difficult experience and, instead of being paralyzed, can transform her pain into a passionate, clear-headed campaign to help others. *Honest Medicine* is a well-written, easy-to-understand look at treatments that have been all but overlooked by the medical world because they are not potential financial blockbusters. But they are potential lifesavers, as Schopick demonstrates in the book's meticulous research and interviews with doctors, patients and advocates who use these treatments in their practices or have personally benefited from them.

—Mary Shomon, *New York Times* bestselling author of
The Thyroid Diet: Manage Your Metabolism for Lasting Weight Loss

One of the themes in Julia's book is her zeal and enthusiasm to change medicine for the better, yet she believes this to be impossible. I would disagree. After living and working in mainstream medicine for forty years, I have seen medicine change. It is continually changing. Join with Julia Schopick and thousands of other health activists demanding these effective treatments ignored by mainstream medicine. A revolution is at hand, and Julia's new book, *Honest Medicine*, is leading the charge with banner held high.

—Jeffrey Dach, MD, author of *Natural Medicine 101*,
and founder of a Hollywood, Florida clinic,
specializing in Bioidentical Hormones and Natural Thyroid

Honest Medicine is a much-needed book in this time of "health care reform." In it, Julia Schopick provides a roadmap for effective solutions to many chronic conditions. Most importantly, the case histories Julia presents in *Honest Medicine* will provide hope to so many people suffering with chronic illnesses, by showing that patients do not have to take toxic pharmaceutical medications that neither treat the underlying cause of their illness nor improve the conditions. I recommend *Honest Medicine* to all who are open-minded and looking for safe, effective therapies that have a sound biochemical basis behind them. This book should be required reading for all physicians and patients searching for safe and effective therapies.

—David Brownstein, MD, Medical Director of the Center for
Holistic Medicine in West Bloomfield, MI, and author of nine books
on integrative medical topics

Rather than merely writing a book, a huge undertaking in itself, Julia Schopick has created a community of men and women who have joined her in presenting potentially lifesaving information in the service of others. The variety of voices sharing their experiences and expertise not only makes the book as easy to read and absorbing as a novel, I felt as if I had made some new friends along the way. These pages are filled with practical advice and information about a group of four treatments whose time has come. In addition to describing these treatments, Julia gives readers a behind-the-scenes look at healthcare as it is today and encourages us to imagine a better future—one individual at a time—until these treatments finally reach full acceptance. Thanks, Julia!

—Virginia McCullough, co-author with Paul Harch, MD,
The Oxygen Revolution

Born out of personal tragedy, Julia Schopick's *Honest Medicine* is a "must read." Run out to get this book and learn how to prevent or even reverse disease with the often unknown, but potentially lifesaving treatments she features. Her outstanding interview with Wellness TalkRadio was life-changing for so many of my listeners. I look forward to many more interviews with Julia regarding "patient-evidence-based treatments," like those she writes about in this wonderful book.

—Kristin Costello, WellnessTalkRadio.com

Well done! Three decades as a physician has left me realizing that there are few illnesses that truly can't be helped. The problem is not lack of effective treatments—but rather a medical system that will only approve and teach about patentable (and therefore very expensive) therapies. When doctors tell you they can't help you, thank them for their honesty. And then read Julia Schopick's book!

—Jacob Teitelbaum, MD, author of the best-selling book,
From Fatigued to Fantastic! (3rd revised edition, Avery/Penguin Group)

Julia Schopick's powerful new book, *Honest Medicine,* is a comprehensive and extremely well-researched work filled with fascinating alternative ways of combating many horrendous diseases that affect millions of people throughout the world. Her medical savvy reigns supreme throughout the book and is conveyed to us in a language that is totally understandable and relatable. Dr. Bernard Bihari, the pioneer of low dose naltrexone for autoimmune diseases, is one of the heroes of Julia's book. He was also my partner for over twenty years. This tender warrior fought so gallantly to make this affordable, non-toxic drug more readily accessible to the public—to patients with autoimmune diseases like multiple sclerosis, HIV/AIDS, fibromyalgia and Crohn's. Julia's splendid book is a marvelous legacy to this remarkable man. I hope that people with autoimmune diseases will read *Honest Medicine.* But I also hope that everyone who has the slightest interest in, or curiosity about, the subject of health and how the immune system functions will read it, as well. Lastly, I want to express my gratitude to Julia for taking the time to care, and also to research and write *Honest Medicine.* Her commitment to getting the word out about LDN and other immune-boosting treatments shines brightly throughout the book.

—Jacqueline L. Young, New York City

HONEST MEDICINE

EFFECTIVE, TIME-TESTED, INEXPENSIVE TREATMENTS FOR LIFE-THREATENING DISEASES

Including Multiple Sclerosis, Epilepsy, Liver Disease, Lupus, Rheumatoid Arthritis and Other Diseases

BY

JULIA SCHOPICK

Innovative Health Publishing

Oak Park, Illinois

HONEST MEDICINE:
EFFECTIVE, TIME-TESTED, INEXPENSIVE TREATMENTS FOR LIFE-THREATENING DISEASES

Including Multiple Sclerosis, Epilepsy, Liver Disease, Lupus, Rheumatoid Arthritis and Other Diseases

ISBN: 978-0-9829690-0-7

Published by:
Innovative Health Publishing
Oak Park, Illinois
www.HonestMedicine.com

Editor: Beth Barany, Barany Consulting
Cover Design: George Foster, Foster Covers
Layout Design: Joel Friedlander, Marin Book Works
Index: Nancy K. Humphreys, Wordmaps

Go to www.HonestMedicine.com for special promotions, premiums and bulk orders.

Dedication

Honest Medicine is gratefully dedicated to

Dr. Bernard Bihari
(November 11, 1931-May 16, 2010)
who changed the lives of many thousands of patients with
autoimmune diseases, HIV/AIDS and many cancers

and to

My husband Tim Fisher
(March 13, 1949-November 8, 2005)
who changed my life forever.

I wish they were both here to read this book.

Table of Contents

Foreword

Compressing the Learning Curve

By Jim Abrahams

Founder, The Charlie Foundation to Help Cure Pediatric Epilepsy

More often than not, when we get really sick, we go to the doctor, we get better, and life goes on.

But sooner or later that's not going to work—for any of us.

My observation is that when it doesn't work, when the doctor doesn't help us get better, we all go through a similar range of emotions. They frequently begin with fear and denial. They can continue through anger, guilt, sadness, distrust, frustration, desperation and any of a number of others. It's human nature. But somewhere along the line, before we decide to throw in the towel, we realize that these feelings are a kind of emotional wheel-spinning, and the instinct to fight kicks in. Nothing necessarily intellectual about the fight. It's a bare knuckle, no-holds-barred, survival-instinct kind of fight. It's a battle we don't know whether we can win.

Despite the uncertainties of undertaking this battle, I believe that the quicker any of us can get from that initial onset of fear to the raw instinct to fight, the better our chance of winning. There's a learning curve involved. It can take weeks, months, even years.

But I also believe that the sooner we make it through that curve, the steeper the slope of the curve, then the sooner we take off the gloves, and the better our chance for good health. The more rapidly we figure out that even the best doctor can be wrong, the faster we realize the uncanny relationship between prescribed treatments and their financial rewards, the quicker we understand the other frailties of our health care system, the sooner we begin to trust our instincts and insist on hard answers, the quicker we learn to take over the reins of our medical destinies, the better off we are.

Eight years ago, I was diagnosed with acute myelogenous leukemia (AML). The first oncologist I saw told me I had a fifty percent chance of surviving for two years. I didn't like the guy—not just for what he was saying. His answers were clipped. His information was abbreviated. His decisions were unilateral. He made me feel like he had more important things to do than explain how and why I was going to die, or what he was going to do about it. (Incidentally, I later found out the treatment he was suggesting would most certainly have killed me.)

But I was lucky. Even at the time, it all felt very familiar to me. I was sensitive to his attitude. My antennae were tuned in. You see, I had been through the learning curve. Ten years earlier when my son Charlie started having epilepsy, we had encountered a similar stone wall. Eventually, after months of a far-too-slow learning curve, Charlie's epilepsy was cured by the Ketogenic Diet. (Read Charlie's story in Chapter 7.)

It turned out the learning curve my family experienced when Charlie was sick saved my life as well as his. But because of his experience we got there much quicker, within days, the second time. And with far less collateral damage. Quite simply, I knew immediately to trust my instincts, put on the gloves and fight. I fired the doctor, and found another who was willing to be a partner in an informed joint decision-making process. The new doctor explained my condition and the options. He listened. He consulted his colleagues. He answered my questions. He gave me reading material. *We* picked a treatment. Here I am.

I think that helping us compress the learning curve is one of the many goals Julia Schopick achieves in her most thorough, informative and inspirational book, *Honest Medicine.* By meticulously chronicling the histories of Low Dose Naltrexone, alpha lipoic acid, the Ketogenic Diet and Silverlon, Julia shares with us not only that there are proven treatments out there that our physicians may not tell us about, but equally importantly, how we can take personal control of our medical destinies.

At the beginning of her book, Julia talks about what those of us who have shared our stories in the book have in common. I would add one other element. We all wish we had learned our lessons earlier. We all wish we had compressed the learning curve. We all wish we had the courage to embrace patient empowerment sooner. The fact that we didn't will forever remain among the battle scars of our lives.

So here's hoping that you will take these valuable messages from *Honest Medicine.* Here's wishing longer, healthier, more self-reliant lives for us all. And here's hoping that somewhere Tim Fisher, Julia's husband, is smiling down on his wife's valiant efforts to bring a further meaning to his life.

Jim Abrahams
Santa Monica, California
August 2010

Preface

Hypnotic Trance

By Burton M. Berkson, MD, MS, PhD

Many doctors, patients and patients' families are in a hypnotic trance when it comes to effective medicine. This statement may come as a surprise to some of you, though if you've picked up Julia Schopick's book, *Honest Medicine*, you may already be aware of this trance. Allow me to explain.

First, let me affirm that certain types of conventional medicine are very effective. For example, antibiotics, trauma surgery, intensive care medicine, and certain cardiology techniques save many lives. However, many other well-accepted and standard medical treatments just don't work. Some modalities, like chemotherapy, when used to treat cancers that are non-responsive to it, just make the patient sicker. Other treatments, such as certain biological response modifiers for rheumatoid arthritis, just mask symptoms, don't improve a person's underlying health, and may incite certain cancers.

As a child, I had a cousin who was a Harvard-educated orthopedic surgeon at the University of Chicago Medical School. My family believed that as a doctor he was beyond reproach. They believed this not because they had evaluated his surgical technique, his bedside manner, or whether his patients were helped by the medical services that he provided to them, but because somebody told them that an Ivy League education was superior to any other education.

As far as my family was concerned, it was taken for granted that my cousin was a better doctor than someone who had trained at a lesser-known, less prestigious state school.

Similar to what they believed made a good doctor, my family believed that there was conventional medicine and then there was medicine that couldn't be trusted. If the treatment was standard of care, it was superior and to be followed; any other course of treatment was quackery. Perhaps they came by these ideas by observing snake oil salesmen take advantage of people who were desperate for a cure. But by thinking this way, they discounted efficacious treatments based on tradition, history and science, if those treatments weren't accepted by the medical mainstream.

It seemed to me that my family was in a hypnotic trance when it came to medicine. They were dazzled by brand-name educations and mainstream medical practices. And if a well-known doctor said a treatment worked, it did—even if it didn't.

Although I was a naturally suspicious person, I didn't break out of my trance until a series of personal experiences led me to question the way medicine was practiced. It all started when I began medical school in Chicago a short time after I graduated from college. I was an immature, anti-authoritarian young man and I didn't take my opportunity to become a doctor seriously. At that time, I didn't want to live the life of a medical doctor. Waking up at five in the morning and knocking myself out in the office all day and at the hospital at night was not what I wanted for my life.

The first block of classes I took in medical school were concerned with anatomy and histology. Medical school at that time was very formal and many students sat at their desks with folded hands, wearing ties. They believed that they were very fortunate to have been admitted to medical school. They just sat there and did not ask many questions.

After class, I would approach the professor to ask questions. It seemed that I was the only one who did this. He told me that at my stage of medical school, I had no questions to ask. He told me that in medical school, the professors lectured on relevant material and the student memorized it. Then during a test, the student would regurgitate the material and pass the test. And if the student did this for four years, he would graduate with an MD. I realized that medical school was no place for independent thought. It was a place where people were *programmed* to think like medical doctors. This wasn't education; it was training.

I wasn't in medical school for very long that time around. I left midway through my first year, partly because I was immature, and partly because I wasn't allowed to think independently. I decided instead to enter graduate school to earn a master's degree in Biology at Eastern Illinois University, and then a PhD in Mycology and Zoology at the University of Illinois. My dissertation was on the cell biology of fungi. Graduate work in the biological sciences at the University of Illinois was a genuine education rather than the training I had experienced in medical school. The students in my department were always encouraged to have new thoughts and to question the status quo. In fact, my major professor made me promise that if in my research I found that he had published something that was incorrect, I would publish a paper stating that he was wrong. To me, that was real science.

As I relay in greater detail in Chapter 4, while I was in graduate school, my wife, Ann, became pregnant and had a miscarriage. When we asked her gynecologist if she would ever be able to have a child, he told us he thought she would have no problems with future pregnancies.

Ann became pregnant again and had another miscarriage. We were both very discouraged. The doctor advised her that multiple miscarriages just happen and that it was very unlikely that she would miscarry again.

At that time I believed that if we changed doctors and went to the head of the department of gynecology at a prestigious university, the outcome would be very different. So that's what we did. The distinguished gynecologist told Ann that with his care, she would be able to carry a baby to term. The next time Ann became pregnant, the pregnancy ended with a miscarriage in the sixth month. The new gynecologist said there was nothing more he could do for us. He had no suggestions or advice, except to get her pregnant again. We were even more disheartened.

In frustration, I went to the medical library at the University of Illinois and spent several hours looking through the gynecological journals. I finally found a relevant article that described a series of cases that were similar to ours, as well as a medical solution to successfully deliver these babies. The article was written by an East Indian doctor, Dr. Vithalrao Nagesh Shirodkar from Goa, India.

I copied the article and brought it to my wife's doctor. He appeared to be insulted. He thought that by this act we were questioning his knowledge of gynecology. He took the article, threw it into the trash, and asked indignantly, "Do I tell you how to do microbiology research?"

In that instant, my medical hypnotic trance was broken. It occurred to me that a doctor who was the head of a department at a prestigious American university was not necessarily more knowledgeable than a doctor practicing in a foreign country. I returned to the library and searched the journals until I found a doctor near us, Dr. Martin Clyman, who could perform the Shirodkar procedure for us.

My wife became pregnant again, and Dr. Clyman, using the Shirodkar procedure, assisted her to carry our baby girl to term, and a successful birth. Five years later we were blessed with another child, a baby boy.

Today the Shirodkar procedure, or cerclage, is the standard approach for correcting the problem my wife had: an incompetent cervical os. But thirty-nine years ago it was considered a type of alternative medicine. It was in reality an innovative idea developed by a doctor in a third world country who was a leader and a thinker rather than a follower.

This experience changed my life and the way I viewed medicine forever. It even propelled me back to medical school to complete my MD. I never thought I would practice medicine, but at least I would be able to advise my family members on medical treatments when they needed them.

Honest Medicine's author, Julia Schopick, a caring and intelligent woman, was also under illusions about what constituted good medicine. When her husband Tim was diagnosed with a devastating cancer of his brain, she was so stunned that she passively allowed the doctors to take over, without questioning them. While today she feels that some of the treatments Tim underwent saved his life, she soon realized that, in many cases, the course of treatment he was advised to take by his well-respected doctors actually made things worse. Then, in 2001, when Tim's suture line wouldn't heal and he developed a head wound, the doctors' treatments—repeated surgeries over the course of ten months—made him worse and worse.

After researching treatment options for Tim, Julia—with advice from Dr. Carlos Reynes, an internal medicine physician, and also a friend—found Silverlon, a cloth patch made from a material containing silver ions. With the consent of Tim's neurosurgeon, she applied the patch to Tim's head and the wound closed.

But even though Tim's wound healed almost instantly, her husband's specialists were not at all interested in learning about

Silverlon. Nor did they accept that this non-standard silver cloth had been what had closed Tim's wound for the first time in months. This behavior by the doctors broke Julia out of her hypnotic trance. She had always been a relentless student and scholar of medical innovation. But now, Julia had a mission to let others know about her experiences and the experiences of those in similar situations to hers, so that they could find efficacious medical solutions more quickly and easily than she had.

Here was something she was certain had worked. There was no doubt in Julia's mind that Silverlon had healed her husband's head wound, literally overnight. The doctors' negative reactions stunned and shocked her. These doctors had failed over and over to heal Tim's head. Yet, they denied that Silverlon had worked. She knew that there was something dangerous going on.

For Julia, if you saw something terrible, you did something about it, in the best way you could. She had to get the story out. She thought, "If this could happen to me—doctors ignoring treatments that worked—how many other people are being affected by such close-minded thinking?"

In Julia's new book, *Honest Medicine*, she describes the work of brave and innovative men and women who have pioneered treatments that have relieved the suffering of thousands upon thousands of people. All of them have tried to communicate their successes to the public and the medical community; all have been essentially ignored or ferociously criticized by people who did not take the time to listen to the sense and the science of the therapies. In some cases, the reason for ignoring or criticizing the treatment was because the listeners were themselves in a medical hypnotic trance. In other cases, it was because an inexpensive and efficacious therapy would potentially damage their lucrative businesses.

In *Honest Medicine*, I've done my part to share the role I've played in bringing attention to non-standard treatments. It has been an honor to be part of this book, and to bring to light these success stories of how innovative and time-tested treatments, often forgotten or ignored by the medical establishment, have improved and even saved people's lives.

As you "follow your gut," as Julia Schopick says, and inform yourself about what has really helped people with difficult-to-treat illnesses, keep in mind that your healthcare is in your hands.

Burton M. Berkson, MD, MS, PhD
Las Cruces, New Mexico
August 2010

Welcome to the World of Low-Cost, Innovative Treatments that Work

CHAPTER 1

It Could Happen to You ...

One early October morning in 1990, a 41-year-old man, Timothy Fisher, underwent brain surgery to remove a life-threatening tumor the size of an orange. Over the next ten years, he endured a series of treatments, chemotherapy, more surgeries, radiation, horrible side effects and complications that changed his life forever.

And mine.

Tim was my husband, and he lived fifteen years post-surgery—twelve years beyond the three years his doctors had originally predicted. We both felt we owed a large portion of his post-surgical longevity and quality of life to lots of non-standard-of-care treatments that included diet and supplements. But in 2001, he had a recurrence of his tumor, and after this surgery, his skin wouldn't heal. Ten months later, it finally did, due entirely to a little-known treatment called Silverlon. But by then, because of the cumulative effect of all the invasive surgical treatments his doctors tried that had failed, Tim was already brain-injured and paralyzed. How I wish we had found Silverlon ten months earlier!

This book is written because of Tim.

And this book is written for you and your loved ones.

Because I want you to find the potentially lifesaving treatments your doctor probably doesn't know about—treatments like those that helped Tim live years beyond his doctors' prognoses—so that you can find them before it's too late.

Because thousands upon thousands of patient success stories about using such treatments show they have a high probability of working. In fact, in many cases, they work far better than the standard-of-care treatments doctors are used to prescribing. More on that in Sections 2 to 4.

Because there are more resources out there than you may know about. Please see all the links in this book and on my website, www.HonestMedicine.com.

And finally, because, frankly, you've got nothing to lose by informing yourself and your loved ones that there may be a better way.

You don't have to take my word for it. Please take some time to visit all the links I share in this book, in the Appendix, and on my website, and study the information for yourself.

A word about the Internet links in this book: *Honest Medicine* is full of resources, many listed as links to websites and to PDFs. Due to the challenge of formatting electronic links in a printed book, you may find it difficult to use these links as published here. If you do, go to http://www.HonestMedicine.com/hyperlinks.html for a complete list. All links were correct at the time of publication.

This book is comprised of several personal stories—stories by patients and medical experts, as well as my own experiences and observations.

The patient and medical expert stories that follow will be of special interest to those of you who have life-threatening diseases, such as multiple sclerosis, rheumatoid arthritis, childhood epilepsy, lupus, liver disease and many other serious conditions—even some cancers. I hope you will also share the true stories in this book with your relatives and friends who have these diseases.

Why Listen to Me?

In addition to this book having a deeply personal meaning to me, I have been an interested and concerned health writer for many years. I've written for *American Medical News*, the AMA publication; *ADVANCE*, the professional publication for physical therapists; *SEARCH*, the National Brain Tumor Foundation newsletter; and *Alternative and Complementary Therapies*, a publication for holistic health practitioners. My work and essays have also been featured in the *British Medical Journal*, *Modern Maturity*, and the *Chicago Sun-Times*. In addition, I have been a public relations professional for the last twenty-plus years. And since Tim's death (and especially for the past three years), I have used my considerable know-how to get the word out about promising but not-so-well-known treatments via my website, www.HonestMedicine.com.

Why I'm Writing This Book

In addition to sharing real-world practical information and stories with you, there is another reason I'm writing this book.

During his long illness, Tim and I both came to believe that the medical profession (or "medical industry," as we often referred to it) was in dire need of change. Naïvely, I vowed to be personally responsible for making some of these changes single-handedly. In fact, one day, I confidently announced, "Before I die, I intend to change the medical system!"

To which Tim replied, with that wonderfully skeptical stare of his, "Jule, you know that's ridiculous." Then he paused, looking quite terrified, and said, "Knowing you, I think you may actually do it!"

I have long ago given up on the idea of changing the medical system. Frankly, I no longer think it's possible. But now, many years after I made that confident (no, arrogant) promise to Tim, I still fervently believe that I can help people by educating them and giving them confidence and knowledge, so that they will be able to change the way they relate to the medical system, and to their doctors.

The truth is that nearly every patient or loved one I've spoken with over the years, including the contributors to this book, has had to face down his or her gut-wrenching fear about confronting doctors, and thus, making them angry. Many times I, too, found myself feeling like a chastised child in front of my husband's doctors. I am grateful that I was finally able to overcome my fear to the point where I could confront Tim's doctors enough to get him better care. I hope that this book will encourage you, my readers, to do the same.

When patients and their families become more knowledgeable and more proactive, I strongly believe they won't need to use this flawed medical system so often; and when they do need to use it, they will be in a more educated, powerful position, and will be able to evaluate and choose treatments for themselves—including treatments like those I feature in this book—even if their doctors don't approve of their choices.

That's what I hope to accomplish with my website, www.HonestMedicine.com, and with this book.

The Focus of This Book: Why These Treatments?

Specifically, this book addresses three treatments, all available in the United States, the United Kingdom and Canada: Intravenous Alpha Lipoic Acid, the Ketogenic Diet and Low Dose Naltrexone. Some of these treatments are also available in other parts of the world, including Italy, Israel, India, Australia and many Asian countries.

In Chapters 2 and 3, I also cover a fourth treatment—Silverlon—mostly to highlight Tim's story. I include this treatment because our experience with it in 2002 exposed me to the bias of conventional doctors against inexpensive, innovative treatments they don't know about—treatments like the ones I am profiling in this book.

People often ask me, "Why are you writing about these particular treatments? What do they have in common?"

My answer: The treatments I found all have similar, very compelling characteristics.

1. They have been around for many years, ranging from "only" twenty-five to over ninety years.

2. These treatments have benefited hundreds, sometimes many thousands, of patients, as documented by many experts.

3. These treatments have all benefited extremely sick patients with life-threatening illnesses ranging from epilepsy to multiple sclerosis, and even HIV/AIDS and cancer. The results have been stunning and documented by the patients (e.g., seizures stopped, MS patients being able to walk, etc.).

4. The treatments all have medical practitioners—and in most cases, MDs—who prescribe the medications, and openly champion them.

5. In most cases, the patients who have benefited from these treatments are extremely passionate about helping others to learn about them. The patients often devote a great deal of their time, mostly unpaid, to holding fundraisers and educating the public.

6. These treatments all work for conditions for which conventional medicine often does not have adequate solutions.

7. And finally, while some are natural treatments, such as diets or supplements, and others are off-label uses of generic drugs, they all have one thing in common: No one is making large amounts of money from these treatments—especially when compared to the amount of money that is made from the treatments championed by the pharmaceutical industry. To back up this fact, I provide links and statistics in the Appendix and throughout the book.

Contributors to This Book

In the following four sections of *Honest Medicine*, you will learn more about the three featured treatments, as seen through the eyes of two groups of people: (a) professionals and (b) patients and their family members. You will discover their missions, and in some cases, their life's work.

Professionals—doctors and dietitians—whose patients have been helped by these treatments:

- Burt Berkson, MD, MS, PhD (Intravenous Alpha Lipoic Acid [ALA] and Low Dose Naltrexone [LDN])
- Millicent Kelly, RD (The Ketogenic Diet)
- Beth Zupec-Kania, RD, CD (The Ketogenic Diet)
- David Gluck, MD (LDN)

and

Patients, and patients' family members, whose lives have been changed, and even saved, because they found one or more of these treatments:

- Jim Abrahams, Ketogenic Diet champion, Founder of The Charlie Foundation to Help Cure Pediatric Epilepsy: http://charliefoundation.org/
- Mary Jo Bean, Intravenous ALA
- Paul Marez, Intravenous ALA and LDN
- Emma Williams, Ketogenic Diet Advocate, Founder of Matthew's Friends, http://site.matthewsfriends.org/
- Jean McCawley, Ketogenic Diet Advocate, Founder of The Stevens Johnson Syndrome Foundation, http://www.sjsupport.org
- Linda Elsegood, LDN Advocate, Founder of the LDN Research Trust, www.LDNResearchTrust.org

- Mary Boyle Bradley, LDN Advocate, author, Internet radio talk show host
- Malcolm West, LDN Advocate, co-founder, LDN Aware, http://LDNaware.org

How to Use This Book

If you are pressed for time, I urge you to start by reading this section, Section 1, so that you'll understand the main point of the book. Then, go to the sections and chapters that are of most interest and relevance to your personal situation.

After you read those sections that have the most relevance to your personal situation, I hope you will then backtrack and read the other sections, too. After learning about some of these other treatments you didn't know about before, you may be surprised to learn that you know other people who might be helped by these treatments. If you do, please pass this book on to them. (Or better yet, buy them a copy!)

How This Book Is Organized

Section 1: Welcome to the World of Low-Cost, Innovative Treatments that Work

Section 1: This section provides an overview of the book—with an introduction, some background and a general synopsis of the treatments I am profiling.

In this chapter (Chapter 1), I give an introduction to the book, including my reasons for writing it and what I hope to accomplish with it. I also include my credentials, the book's focus, an introduction to the treatments I am profiling, and why I chose them. You'll meet the people whose stories I include and my reasons for choosing each one. The concept of patient-based evidence is introduced and explained here, as well.

In Chapter 2, I tell Tim's story, to share with you how my love for him led me to do online research to find out-of-the-box treatments that extended his life. Here, I concentrate especially on the dramatic way in which I found Silverlon, the product that closed up Tim's non-healing suture line, literally overnight. As you read Chapter 2, I hope you will realize that it is also possible for you to find similar treatments that work, especially when it becomes obvious that your doctors are not finding successful resolutions to your medical problems, or to those of a loved one.

Chapter 3 tells the rest of our personal story, about how our doctors responded to our experience with Silverlon with an almost total lack of interest. You'll see how stunned and upset I was by their negative reactions. It was my first personal experience with this kind of uncurious response of doctors to learning about treatments they hadn't learned about in the traditional way—i.e., from medical school or medical journals. Most importantly, our experience with Silverlon provided my motivation for writing this book.

Finally, in Chapter 3, I describe how I chose the other three treatments that form the crux of this book.

Section 2: Intravenous Alpha Lipoic Acid

Section 2: An intravenous antioxidant therapy, also known as lipoic acid; a naturally occurring compound. Its therapeutic uses include diabetes, atherosclerosis, neurodegenerative disorders, liver diseases, and other conditions. (http://www.umm.edu/altmed/articles/alpha-lipoic-000285.htm)

Intravenous Alpha Lipoic Acid was pioneered by Dr. Burt Berkson (MD, MS, PhD); he first used it in the 1970s for regenerating organs, especially livers.

In Chapter 4, Dr. Berkson tells his story in his own words: how he went against his hospital superiors, who were upset with him because the treatment he was using was not "standard of care." (http://en.wikipedia.org/wiki/Standard_of_care#Medical_standard_of_care)

In addition to Dr. Berkson's contribution to this book, two of his patients have written chapters. In Chapter 5, Mary Jo Bean tells how her combination of two liver diseases—hepatitis C and cirrhosis—would have killed her, if she hadn't found out about Dr. Berkson. And in Chapter 6, Paul Marez describes how his Stage IV pancreatic cancer was cured by Dr. Berkson. Both patients had been given a death sentence by their conventional doctors. Neither patient had been medically sophisticated beforehand. Yet both Mary Jo and Paul were determined not to die, and therefore, found the wisdom and curiosity to look beyond the advice of their conventional doctors. They both found Dr. Berkson; they are both alive today.

Section 3: The Ketogenic Diet

According to Epilepsy.com, "The Ketogenic Diet is a special high-fat, low-carbohydrate diet that helps to control seizures in some people with epilepsy. It is prescribed by a physician and carefully monitored by a dietitian." (http://www.epilepsy.com/epilepsy/treatment_ketogenic_diet)

In Section 3, I focus on the Ketogenic Diet, which has cured tens of thousands of children of their seizures for over ninety years at Johns Hopkins and other prominent medical institutions. However, in the 1940s, with the advent of anti-seizure medications, its use declined considerably.

Then in 1994, Hollywood film writer/director/producer Jim Abrahams became the diet's champion, soon after it stopped his infant son Charlie's seizures within forty-eight hours. This, after many medications, and even one surgery, failed to have any effect.

Jim created The Charlie Foundation to Help Cure Pediatric Epilepsy to spread the word about the diet: http://www.charlie foundation.org. Thanks to Jim and The Charlie Foundation, numerous hospitals in the United States and around the world are using the diet today. And thousands and thousands of children are now seizure-free.

Jim contributed Chapter 7 and the Foreword to this book. And together, dietitians Millicent Kelly and Beth Zupec-Kania contributed Chapter 8. Their hard work and dedication have also helped to keep the diet alive.

Lastly, two parents share their unique stories about using the Ketogenic Diet with their children, both of whom were plagued with intractable forms of childhood epilepsy. In Chapter 9, Emma Williams describes her six-year battle to convince doctors in the UK to let her try the Ketogenic Diet for her son Matthew. Year after year, they turned her down, telling her that drugs were the best way to treat him. Sadly, because of years of seizures—and perhaps partly because of the side effects of the drugs themselves—by the time Matthew was put on the diet, he was already severely brain injured. He remains so today. However, the diet reduced the number of Matthew's seizures so greatly that Emma is able to keep him at home with her, rather than having to put him in a residential home. She created an organization called Matthew's Friends to spread the word about the diet in the UK, so that other parents would be able to find it early in their quest for answers. (http://site. matthewsfriends.org) Emma is convinced that if Matthew had been put on the diet years earlier, he wouldn't be brain injured today.

In Chapter 10, Jean McCawley tells a similar story about her daughter Julie—except that Jean found the diet while Julie was still an infant. Unfortunately, before she found it, Julie had already been irreparably damaged by Phenobarbital, the very first anti-convulsant medication doctors gave the baby to stop her seizures.

Anti-convulsants and other medications can cause a rare disease called Stevens Johnson Syndrome. In Julie's case, SJS caused her skin to peel off and left her blind in one eye, and nearly blind in the other. (Click on "Julie's Story" at http://charliefoundation.org under the photo of Meryl Streep.) Jean has created a not-for-profit organization, The Stevens Johnson Syndrome Foundation, to educate parents about this debilitating and life-threatening condition, which she believes is much more common than doctors like to admit. (http://sjsupport.org) She is also deeply involved in educating other parents about the Ketogenic Diet, so that they won't suffer the way she and Julie did.

Section 4: Low Dose Naltrexone (LDN)

Low Dose Naltrexone: The drug naltrexone, used in doses approximately one-tenth the dose prescribed for drug/alcohol rehabilitation purposes, is being used as an "off-label" treatment for certain immunologically related disorders. The use of LDN for such diseases as cancer was first proposed by Ian Zagon, PhD, and LDN's broader clinical effects in humans were proposed by Bernard Bihari, MD. (For more on LDN see http://en.wikipedia.org/wiki/Low_dose_ naltrexone. For a definition of "off-label," see http://en.wikipedia.org/ wiki/Off-label_use.)

While working with drug addicts in Brooklyn in the 1980s, Harvard-educated neurologist, Bernard Bihari, MD, discovered that a very low-dose, off-label use of the drug, naltrexone, could be used just as successfully to modulate the immune system. At a much higher dose, naltrexone had already been approved by the FDA to get addicts off drugs. Used at a very low dose, naltrexone was able to stop the progression of such autoimmune diseases as MS, lupus, rheumatoid arthritis, Crohn's disease, and even HIV/ AIDS and some cancers.

Since the 1980s, LDN has become a cause célèbre. So much so, that many of the patients who take LDN, and their family members, have written books. For instance:

- *The Promise of Low Dose Naltrexone Therapy: Potential Benefits in Cancer, Autoimmune, Neurological and Infectious Disorders* by MS patient, SammyJo Wilkinson and medical writer, Elaine Moore (http://www.amazon.com/Promise-Low-Dose-Naltrexone-Therapy/dp/0786437154)

- *Up the Creek With a Paddle: Beat MS and Many Autoimmune Disorders with Low Dose Naltrexone* by Mary Boyle Bradley (http://www.amazon.com/Creek-Paddle-Autoimmune-Disorders-Naltrexone/dp/1413765998)

LDN patients have also raised money to fund studies, as have some doctors. None of these people are getting vast sums of money for their efforts, which makes them unique in the conventional medical landscape, where "follow the money" is so often the rule.

Three patients and one physician have contributed their stories to this section. In Chapter 11, Dr. David Gluck, Dr. Bihari's childhood friend and colleague, gives us his take on the importance of LDN to the world of medicine. MS patient Linda Elsegood (Chapter 12) tells how her difficult journey to finding LDN led her to create the UK charity, the LDN Research Trust, in order to fund research and help other patients find LDN more easily than she had. And in Chapter 13, Mary Boyle Bradley tells the dramatic story of how she found LDN for her husband Noel, and how she, too, became determined to spread the word.

Finally, in Chapter 14, Malcolm West describes how he used the toxic pharmaceutical drugs his doctors prescribed for many years, only to have his multiple sclerosis get progressively worse. Finally, he became so ill that he lost his job, and with it, his health insurance. Malcolm had to find a less expensive treatment. So he went online and found LDN. Almost immediately, his MS improved—

and very dramatically, at that. He, too, has become a most enthusiastic and vocal LDN advocate. With other LDN advocates, he has created an umbrella website that contains information about the use of LDN throughout the world: http://LDNaware.org.

In all three cases, these patients' doctors discouraged them from using LDN. Also, like the other contributors to this book, all three of these patient advocates wish they had found this treatment sooner.

Why These Champions?

People often ask me what characteristics these champions share in common. I have thought long and hard about how to put into words what I have always intuitively known.

First, all these champions have as their mission to get the message out about treatments that have saved many, many lives.

Second, not one of these professionals and patients—most of whom are now volunteer advocates for the treatments—makes a huge profit from them. Their primary motivation is to help others who need these treatments to find them.

Third, these champions all followed their instincts, even when their superiors, colleagues or physicians told them that their successes with the treatments they were championing were "only anecdotal."

In other words, with all three of these treatments, my heroes would not let people keep dying or get worse by using the standard-of-care treatments their other doctors were encouraging them to use.

For example, instead of following his superiors' orders, Dr. Berkson (Chapter 4) decided to go his own way, and cure more people of end-stage liver disease outside institutional medicine than he ever would have been allowed to cure if he had remained within the university setting. Dr. Berkson saw with his own eyes that, with his treatments, patients were outliving the time they had been given by their doctors. He saw that the first patients he treated with intravenous ALA, Eunice and John Goostree, recovered from their terminal liver disease, as did many, many patients after them. Dr. Berkson wrote articles about these successes, including one article with Dr. Fred Bartter from the National Institutes of Health (NIH), in which seventy-five out of seventy-nine patients with end-stage liver disease got better. (http://honestmedicine.typepad. com/BERKSON-1980-amanitin.pdf)

Jim Abrahams (Chapter 7), too, learned to trust and follow his own instincts, over the advice of his son Charlie's doctors, all of whom were well-known leaders in the field of pediatric epilepsy. Jim saw with his own eyes that the Ketogenic Diet worked for Charlie. He soon learned that the Ketogenic Diet worked better than drugs for countless other children, too.

Jim's instincts also led him to do more research. He uncovered the fact that when one anti-seizure medication doesn't work, the chances are greatly diminished that other drugs will work. This led him to question why Charlie's pediatric neurologist had been trained to try one drug, two drugs, then three, five, nine, even twelve (and some in combination), before trying something "anecdotal" like the Ketogenic Diet. Yet, even this neurologist had to know, from his training, that after the first anti-seizure drug, and then the second, these drugs became less and less effective. It is still a mystery to me why he discouraged Jim from having Charlie try the diet. And Jim has told me recently that he heard this same doctor tell a marketing representative for a seizure medication, "We're still waiting to see …" if the Ketogenic Diet works. This is fifteen years after he saw that the diet worked for Charlie.

This didn't make sense to Jim. And it doesn't make sense to me either.

Training Versus Education: How Conventional Doctors Are Different

But within the conventional medical culture, it does make sense. I think it has something to do with this doctor's (and all doctors') training which, it turns out, teaches them to distrust their own instincts. In Chapter 4, Dr. Berkson points out that doctors are trained, rather than educated, because education requires a certain amount of curiosity about new things, while training requires the retention and repetition of facts. In the atmosphere of medical training that Burt Berkson describes, it takes a lot of courage for doctors to trust what they see, rather than what they were taught.

Just look at some of the more conventional doctors my contributors and I describe in upcoming chapters. Even though they saw that patients were getting better with LDN, they still refused to prescribe it. Similarly, even though other doctors knew that children were doing well with the Ketogenic Diet, they often refused to acknowledge it.

In the end, I have decided that something very important must be trained out of students in medical school, and it has to do with curiosity, with trusting one's instincts. Going a step further, I believe they are literally trained to *distrust* their own instincts, and trust only what they were taught.

The Time Is Right

Unfortunately, every single person featured in this book had to find these treatments on their own. Because these treatments are not considered standard of care—and are not manufactured by large pharmaceutical companies—the patients had to find them without any help from their doctors.

Fortunately, for many reasons, I think that the time is finally right for these treatments to find greater acceptance. And I hope this book will play a significant role in causing that to happen. One of the main reasons the time is right is that, for the last several years, the pharmaceutical industry's duplicity has been making headlines. To me, this is corroboration of my belief that the public is finally ready to listen to what I, and many others, have to say.

There have been numerous media exposés about pharmaceutical companies:

- Rigging the so-called studies, which they themselves fund

- Hiding the results of those studies that actually prove their products don't work

- Heavily publicizing the studies that demonstrate their products' successes

- Hiring the researchers to conduct the studies, making it very clear to them exactly what kinds of results they are expecting the studies to show

- Hiring writers to write the articles that appear in the medical journals the doctors read

- Hiring big-name doctors—who have done very little, if any, of the actual writing—to affix their names to these studies

On HonestMedicine.com, there are many articles attesting to these duplicitous activities that are routinely carried out by pharmaceutical companies. The site also contains thirty-seven articles I have selected for patients to share with their doctors. See http://www.honestmedicine.com/2008/08/financial-ties-between-big-pharma-and-the-medical-establishment-36-selected-articles-published-between-2005-and-2008.html.

I knew the time was finally right for this book when, in April 2008, the *Journal of the American Medical Association (JAMA)* published three articles exposing duplicitous behavior by Merck

Pharmaceuticals. *JAMA* exposed the fact that Merck had engaged in such behavior in the marketing of Vioxx prior to 2004, when Vioxx was pulled from the market. *JAMA* revealed that Merck had engaged in every one of the unsavory practices mentioned above.

Here are the three *JAMA* articles:

1. "Guest Authorship and Ghostwriting in Publications Related to Rofecoxib," by Joseph S. Ross, MD, MHS; Kevin P. Hill, MD, MHS; David S. Egilman, MD, MPH; Harlan M. Krumholz, MD, SM http://jama.ama-assn.org/cgi/content/abstract/299/15/1800

2. "Reporting Mortality Findings in Trials of Rofecoxib for Alzheimer Disease or Cognitive Impairment," by Bruce Pasty, MD, PhD; Richard A. Kronmal, PhD http://jama.ama-assn.org/cgi/content/abstract/299/15/1813

3. "Impugning the Integrity of Medical Science: The Adverse Effects of Industry Influence," by Catherine D. DeAngelis, MD, MPH and Phil B. Fontanarosa, MD, MBA http://jama.ama-assn.org/cgi/content/extract/299/15/1833

For me, the fact that *JAMA* published these three articles exposing Merck's unscrupulous behavior exhibited a huge change in "how things are done." Just two years earlier, in July 2006, *JAMA* itself was exposed by the *Wall Street Journal* for publishing and promoting a flawed study by medical researchers with some very questionable pharmaceutical connections. (See my three-part article, "The JAMA Controversy," at http://www.honestmedicine.com/new_series.)

So, in April 2008, it became clear to me that something new was afoot in the world of pharmaceutical company exposés. The medical journals themselves were beginning to expose duplicity within the pharmaceutical industry.

Because of the media attention given to this kind of questionable behavior, and also because of many excellent, best-selling books about it—such as John Abramson, MD's *Overdosed America*, Marcia Angell, MD's *The Truth About the Drug Companies*, Jay Cohen, MD's *Over Dose: The Case Against the Drug Companies*, and medical journalist, Melody Petersen's *Our Daily Meds*—I feel confident that our country is finally ready to be open to the treatments I am writing about (and others like them), even though they may not have multi-million-dollar, pharmaceutical company-funded studies behind them. I think the public finally understands that such pharmaceutical company-funded "studies" do not necessarily result in safe, effective treatments.

For all the above reasons, I am confident the time is right for this book. I hope that those of you who are reading these patient stories now will pass the information along to any family members and friends who you believe might be helped by reading these personal accounts. Those that can be helped include people with:

- liver diseases;
- autoimmune diseases and cancer; and
- children with intractable epilepsy.

Unfortunately, their friends and family will not likely learn about these treatments from their doctors. But they *can* learn about them from you, and from this book, and its many resources.

Patient-Based Evidence

Personal accounts like these of successful treatments are not "anecdotal." These treatments are backed by evidence provided by numerous patients: real people who have been helped by these treatments. And in the case of the treatments I feature in this book, thousands and thousands of patients have provided the evidence.

This is what I'd like you to understand by the time you've finished reading this book. Unfortunately, far too many doctors dismiss treatments like these, calling them "anecdotal," because they have not been subjected to what they consider to be the gold standard of medical research, i.e., randomized double-blind clinical trials.

In my opinion, this displaced respect is indeed unfortunate, because, as many writers, like John Abramson, MD have observed, pharmaceutical companies, rather than the government, conduct most of today's clinical trials on their own drugs. And even in government-funded studies, there has been evidence of medical researchers with financial ties to pharmaceutical companies.

Given all this—which I call the "dirty big secret" of the pharmaceutical industry's involvement in clinical trials—it's time we gave more respect to patient-based evidence, to which this book is devoted. In my opinion, patient-based evidence may well be the only kind of evidence that is not tainted. By "not tainted," I mean that these patients whose stories are in this book are giving honest appraisals of their personal successes with these treatments. No one is paying them to say anything—unlike the celebrities who are paid huge amounts of money by pharmaceutical companies to hawk their medications.

Patient-Evidence-Based Treatments

When referring to the treatments themselves, I refer to them as patient-evidence-based treatments. It is my sincere hope that by profiling important treatments in this book—treatments that have patient-based evidence to back them up—many more patients will find them, and will be helped.

Who This Book Is For

One last word before we move on: This book is not about exposing all pharmaceutical treatments as bad or ineffective. Many aren't. And this book is not about how alternative treatments are always better than pharmaceutical products. Again, many aren't. And this book is not for people who listen to and follow every word their doctor says as gospel, or for people who listen to other people more than to their own gut. This book is not for them.

Rather, this book is for people who are discerning, who are open to doing their own research (or having someone they trust do it), who are open to being curious, and who are open to new information. This book is also for people who have chronic and life-threatening conditions that have not been helped by the conventional, standard-of-care treatments their doctors have prescribed for them. And this book is for those who realize that medicine should be patient-oriented, not profit-oriented.

Many times, I meet people who seem to think, "There is no other way. If there was an answer, my doctor would know about it." I hope that, after reading this book, you'll know that "It ain't necessarily so!" There may well be many excellent treatments out there that your doctor does not know about. So, let's get started now by looking at four of them.

CHAPTER 2

Our Story: Silverlon and Surgery, Our Search for Healing

In this chapter, based on an article first published by the National Brain Tumor Foundation in their newsletter, *SEARCH*, Winter 2003, Issue 54, and adapted for this book, you'll learn the true story of our success with Silverlon. (http://honest medicine.typepad.com/National-Brain-Tumor-Foundation-Article.pdf)

This article formed the genesis of my mission to get the word out to the public about lifesaving treatments that are not yet accepted by the medical establishment, like the ones highlighted in this book: Silverlon, Intravenous Alpha Lipoic Acid, the Ketogenic Diet and Low Dose Naltrexone.

For ten years, we were lucky and we knew it. My husband Tim was one of the fortunate long-term brain tumor survivors. Although he seemed to suffer all the complications and side effects from his first surgery and subsequent chemotherapy and radiation treatments in 1990 and 1991, he was able to maintain the most important thing: his Self. And we maintained our wonderful marriage in every sense, a full one hundred percent partnership.

One of the best things about Tim's level of survivorship was that, although he was able to work less and less, he could still fully enjoy his two great passions (besides me, of course!): music and reading. In fact, his tumor-forced semi-retirement gave him the opportunity to indulge these passions with no guilt and all pleasure. "Someday," he'd tell me, "I may not be able to enjoy my passions—so I'll enjoy them now."

I happily agreed and became the primary breadwinner, working out of our large apartment and taking numerous breaks throughout the day to talk, cuddle with him, and listen to his lengthy and passionate dissertations about music.

Like all brain tumor families, we knew our time together might be shortened, so we learned to live in the present. At times, we talked about what might happen in the future. We bargained on possible tumor recurrence, or brain damage, as the side effects from his course of whole brain radiation became more and more debilitating.

We did not know that, in the end, it would be Tim's fragile skin, weakened by repeated radiation treatments and surgeries, that would be his Waterloo. When the shoe finally dropped, it nearly toppled us.

What happened to Tim can happen easily to so many brain tumor survivors who undergo post-surgical radiation treatment. I am now passing on what I have learned to other brain tumor survivors, in hopes that long-term survivors will not be toppled by these complications and side effects, and will instead turn into permanent survivors, with a great quality of life.

But first, some background:

In October 1990, 41-year-old Tim underwent surgery to remove a huge, grade 3 astrocytoma from his left frontal lobe. About a month later, he underwent whole brain radiation. For the first four years after that, he seemed to suffer from every possible side effect and complication of both the surgery and the radiation.

These complications caused him to require some eight or nine additional surgeries over the next four years. In addition, from 1990 to 2001, there were several adjustments in his medications, as well as a stroke (another "side effect" of the radiation), infrequent seizures, and numerous trips to the hospital. But finally, we thought we had come out on the other side.

Then, in January 2000, he started having grand mal seizures that wouldn't quit. He was hospitalized for nearly a month in our local community hospital. Although the MRI at the local hospital turned up "nothing unusual," we were understandably tense as we waited for the results of a second MRI in April 2000.

Our neurosurgeon, who had performed the 1990 surgery, said there was "something" on the scan. That "something" was a tumor. He advised having surgery as soon as possible. But, having lived through all the complications and side effects from the first surgery, we weren't keen on the prospect of another. We decided to wait.

After fourteen months, the doctor was adamant about surgery. The tumor was getting dangerously close to Tim's motor strip. In the weeks that followed, I talked back and forth with his nurse, who seemed confident that all the necessary pieces were in place—including having a plastic surgeon to close Tim up because, years ago, Tim's skin had had trouble healing.

The surgery was performed on June 26, 2001. The surgeon (our primary neurosurgeon's partner) greeted us confidently at 7:30 a.m.—and in Tim went.

He came out hours later in almost perfect shape. A miracle! I applauded myself for all the organic food and supplements I'd poured into him over the past five years. Tim was released from the hospital after four days—highly unusual for someone with his history. For one month, everything was perfect.

No changes at all, neurological or physical. We took long walks, went to the movies and out to dinner. Friends came over and Tim would hold court, playing his beloved classical music for them and interpreting it for his various "audiences."

I was astounded and grateful. We were surely blessed.

Then, it happened. The first shoe dropped. We had been trying not to notice a small "spot" on the suture line that seemed slow to heal. The visiting nurses didn't seem to be overly worried, either, so we remained calm. But suddenly, Tim became confused and incontinent—and very soon, I knew we were in deep trouble.

A trip to the emergency room where he'd had surgery a month earlier revealed that air had flooded Tim's brain. After ten hours in the ER, they finally sewed up the tiny holes they found in the suture line where the original incision had been made months earlier. Then they put him on several IV antibiotics at once.

When there's air in the brain, we were told, infection can be assumed. We all hoped the wound would heal, and that we'd be lucky. We weren't. Again, about three weeks later, air flooded his brain. They operated again, this time removing his plastic plate and shunt, and putting him on yet more antibiotics. After three months, he came home.

Tim did extremely well for two months and began to walk again with a walker. We even went out for our sixteenth wedding anniversary, with Tim's caregiver sitting a few feet away. Again we thought we were blessed.

Then, the other shoe dropped. Tim again became disoriented, and this time he had a fever. Since we had been so dissatisfied with the treatment he received in the first hospital, we had found another hospital—and another neurosurgeon.

I took Tim to this hospital for another three-plus months of surgeries to try to fix the suture line, where he had been opened up for the operation. By now, they were putting in external drains on a regular basis, but nothing worked.

Tim's new neurosurgeon was puzzled and "distraught" about Tim's situation. Now the dura (the covering of the brain) was leaking. Meanwhile, I was spending hours and hours online, looking for out-of-the-box treatments that the doctors might not have thought of. I prepared a 200-page report on my findings for the doctors to read. I was to find out later that his doctors hadn't read it, although they had promised that they would.

I tried to get Tim approved for hyperbaric oxygen, which has been known to do wonders for both radiation necrosis and non-healing wounds. But the doctor who ran the chamber at this hospital refused. He was afraid Tim was too fragile. I, too, was afraid, because I just knew Tim was dying.

And I think he would have died, if I hadn't been blessed to be interviewing an Oak Park (Illinois) internist, Carlos Reynes, MD, on behalf of one of my clients. We chatted about personal matters and when he asked, "How's your husband?" I told him. He asked me if I had ever heard of Silverlon. "Silver what?" I inquired. He explained that Silverlon was a healing system comprised of pieces of material made with silver ions which, when wet, caused many of the worst non-healing wounds to heal.

He had used it successfully on several patients with non-healing diabetic wounds. And it was FDA-approved, which meant it had passed all tests for safety.

Dr. Reynes gave me the contact information for the company's sales representatives. I contacted them, and they came to the house, showed me the product, and explained how it worked. I had more questions, so they gave me the name and phone number of the physician who invented the product, Bart Flick, MD. I called him immediately. Dr. Flick asked me to fax him Tim's medical history, which I did. Once he was convinced that Silverlon would work to heal Tim's wound, he agreed to talk with Tim's doctor.

I called Tim's neurosurgeon, only to find out that Tim's head was leaking yet again. "I don't really want to do any more surgery," he said, sounding almost sick. "Tim's been through much too much already."

"Would you consider trying something a bit different?" I asked.

"Yes," he said.

So while I had him hold, I dialed Dr. Flick's number, hoping to place an instant three-way call. Thank goodness, Dr. Flick was there—and available.

Hands shaking, I patched the conference call together and the two doctors spoke, with me quietly crossing all fingers and toes. I heard Dr. Flick offer to supply all the Silverlon dressings for Tim free of charge. That night the samples were on Tim's head. To my knowledge, Tim was the first person to have Silverlon used on a non-healing post-surgical head wound.

That was the last day his head leaked.

To my surprise (shock, really), Tim's doctors did not seem to be at all impressed—or frankly, even interested—in our success with Silverlon. In fact, they all warned me that it might have been a fluke. In any case, they were quite sure it was "anecdotal."

But I really was, and still am, absolutely positive it wasn't a fluke. In fact, Silverlon certainly is a wonderful example of what I now call a patient-evidence-based treatment. Naïvely, I hoped that Tim's success with Silverlon would be repeated many times over for other brain tumor patients with non-healing wounds in the years to come. It didn't happen. Today, I am still hoping that, at some point in the future, one neurosurgeon who hears our story will become excited about Silverlon, and will agree to use it on brain tumor patients' heads. Maybe one will even conduct a trial. Unfortunately, so far, this hasn't happened. I am hoping this book may provide the necessary impetus.

After many talks with Dr. Flick, I understood why Silverlon works—as well as why some doctors are so skeptical. You see, the principle of Silverlon is very different from what doctors learn in medical school about how skin heals. And remember, as I pointed out in the introduction, doctors are trained not to think outside the box, or to be curious. We certainly experienced this lack of *both* curiosity *and* outside-the-box thinking.

Dr. Flick told me he thinks Silverlon helped to heal Tim's head by changing the electrical environment, or electrostatic field, on the surface of the body (i.e., on the skin). He hypothesized that this, in turn, affected the electrical characteristics of the dura mater—the layer surrounding the brain—allowing it to heal. He also told me that silver foils were routinely used as surgical dressings at the prestigious Johns Hopkins University Hospital before antibiotics were invented. So, as it turns out, a variation of Silverlon was in use many years ago.

Dr. Flick told me that he has found, from twenty-plus years of research, that skin has a definite electrical potential. When there is a wound, the electrical potential of the affected area becomes abnormal. He pointed out that if you can pull electrical potential from the surrounding healthier skin, you can reestablish the normal electrical potential at the wound's site. This causes the affected skin to heal more quickly. This is the power of conductive fabrics made from silver.

Silverlon cannot just be placed over the affected area of the skin. In order to harness the electrical potential of healthy skin, the material must be placed wet over the affected area—and it must also touch two centimeters beyond the affected area on all sides. (You can learn more about Silverlon at http://www.silverlon.com.)

I am convinced that if we had known about Silverlon just ten months earlier, it would have given Tim a much better chance of healing from the June 2001 surgery. If we had found Silverlon earlier, I will even go so far as to say that I believe Tim might be alive today.

While I can't be sure that is true, I definitely believe that, if we had found Silverlon earlier, Tim would not have been left with the cognitive deficits he had for the last three-and-a-half years of his life. When he finally came home with me, he was bedbound, incontinent, and nearly paralyzed. So I wrote my article in *SEARCH*, and I am writing my book today, for Tim, in hopes that one day soon, all patients will be able to use treatments like Silverlon that have such convincing patient-based evidence to back them up.

CHAPTER 3

The Rest of Our Silverlon Story: Skepticism and Disbelief

In this chapter, you'll learn "the rest of the story," i.e., how Tim's doctors, and many other doctors who read our story in *SEARCH*, were skeptical about our success with Silverlon, and refused to use it on other brain tumor patients with non-healing post-surgical head wounds.

When my article about our experience with Silverlon was published by the National Brain Tumor Foundation, it created quite a stir among brain tumor patients and their families throughout the country and abroad.

In that article, I was very careful to keep my recounting of our story upbeat, in hopes that doctors who read it would be eager to learn about Silverlon, and possibly use it on some of their non-healing, post-surgical brain tumor patients' heads. (This kind of non-healing suture line—especially in cases where the patient's skin has been previously radiated—is more common than most neuro-surgeons like to admit.)

But, I also knew that if I were to tell the whole "rest of our story" in that article—the part I am telling now—it would be too controversial, and hence, would never have been published. So, in the published article, I purposely neglected to write about how:

- All the extra surgeries had left Tim extremely brain injured, so that when he came home, he was paralyzed, bed-bound, incontinent, and had major memory loss.

And I also decided not to tell about:

- How not one of Tim's doctors was even remotely interested in learning about the treatment that had saved Tim and kept him from dying.

And there was more that I left out of the article, including that the residents (the doctors in training at the hospital), who had liked me very much before this incident, began acting very differently toward me afterwards—suspicious, even cold.

One resident, my favorite, stopped me in the hall. "I've been thinking," he said. "I just don't believe it was the treatment you found that healed Tim's head."

I asked what he thought had done the trick.

"Vancomycin," he intoned with respect—with near reverence, even awe—naming the high-powered IV antibiotic that Tim had already been on for over six weeks, along with several other very expensive IV antibiotics.

I mentioned this fact to him.

His answer—I will never forget it: "Vanco is like that. It kicks in."

Try as I might, I could not interest even one of these residents, or the attending neurosurgeon, in reading any of the materials I had brought to the hospital about Silverlon. I even tried to share with them the FDA reports stating that Silverlon was safe for use on any non-healing wound. In fact, Silverlon was approved by the FDA in 1998 for all non-healing wounds. (For more information, see http://www.silverlon.com/fda.html.) They could not have been less interested. Not one doctor, or resident, read even one of the articles. A few actually told me that their "plates were full."

Thinking back, I don't blame Tim's doctors for not knowing about Silverlon, and therefore, for repeatedly operating on Tim's frayed, previously radiated skin. I don't blame them, because repeated surgeries were the only treatments his doctors knew about. While it makes me very sad to admit this, repeated surgeries in situations like Tim's were, and still are, considered the standard of care. Somehow, surgeons hope that, through these repeated surgeries, they will finally find two pieces of skin that will hold together. Far too many times they don't, and the patient dies.

I do thank his doctors for *allowing* me to use Silverlon on Tim's head while he was in the hospital—even though it was not standard of care for Tim's particular condition.

However, I do blame them for not being even the slightest bit interested in the fact that the Silverlon worked—and that it worked like a miracle for Tim. I also blame them (or, perhaps, I blame the way they were trained) for concluding that our success with Silverlon was probably "anecdotal," and that it was more likely their own treatments (e.g., vancomycin) that miraculously "kicked in" on the very day Silverlon was placed on Tim's head!

By not being interested in the miracle that was achieved for Tim by using this patient-evidence-based treatment, I believe his doctors are preventing their colleagues from learning about a very valuable, lifesaving treatment. They are also responsible, to my way of thinking, for letting lots of other patients like Tim die of their non-healing, previously radiated suture lines. Because, if we had not found Silverlon, Tim would have died then. And I am quite sure his doctors knew it.

Although the doctors at the hospital where Tim's skin healed hadn't seemed interested or curious about our success with Silverlon, I naïvely hoped that some more curious doctors outside of Chicago might be.

The day *SEARCH* began reaching people's homes, distraught family members started calling me from hospitals across the country. "My brother's head is leaking." "My sister's head won't heal." Others sent me emails from foreign countries—all describing similar problems with non-healing post-surgical suture lines.

I convinced the inventor of Silverlon, Bart Flick, MD, who by now had become our friend, to talk with these patients' family members, to offer to speak with their doctors, and to provide Silverlon free of charge for the patients. He agreed, and in at least one case that I know of, he sent the Silverlon to the hospital by overnight mail.

Imagine my surprise when not one of these patients' neurosurgeons wanted to speak with Dr. Flick. And not one agreed to let their leaking, dying patients use this product in lieu of, or even in addition to, surgery.

For three-and-a-half years after Tim came home, I dedicated myself to taking care of him, and to filling out forms and pleading with government personnel to obtain financial coverage through the State of Illinois Brain Injury Waiver Program. After a year, we were finally approved to receive the caregiver services we so desperately needed, so that Tim could be taken care of at home while I worked. (I paid for a caregiver out of pocket for the year before we were approved.) I also kept my home-based public relations business afloat so that I could afford to keep Tim at home.

Even though he was very disabled, he was still Tim, and we were able to have some wonderful times. Several of his friends and I tell about some of those wonderful times in my tribute to Tim, which I wrote on the second anniversary of his death: http://www.honestmedicine.com/2007/11/timothy-mark-fi.html.

Tim died in November 2005. For quite some time after his death, I couldn't help thinking about our difficulties in dealing with the healthcare system. In 2006, I decided to create my Honest

Medicine website in Tim's memory, and in his honor, as my way of educating others about the flaws in our medical system. I also wanted to inform people about other promising (and often lifesaving) treatments like Silverlon, which I was pretty sure their doctors wouldn't tell them about.

But "the rest of the story" about our Silverlon experience also kept gnawing at me. I kept asking myself these questions about Silverlon and other similar treatments:

- Why weren't our doctors—and the other doctors who read about our success with Silverlon—even interested in reading about it, much less willing to consider trying it? (Remember, it was FDA-approved for all non-healing wounds.)

- Were there other similar, lifesaving treatments—like Silverlon—that doctors also weren't telling their patients about? Treatments that were quietly saving lives—once patients themselves searched for and discovered them on their own—but were being under-publicized, or not publicized at all?

- Why aren't these treatments better known? In other words, what is it about our medical system—and our doctors, in particular—that makes them so resistant to learning about (not to mention, trying) anything that is different, no matter how promising? I've often wondered whether these doctors have forgotten their Hippocratic Oath, and if so, how that has happened.

Because of our experience with Silverlon, one lifesaving, patient-evidence-based treatment, I decided to write this book about several treatments that save lives, but that, like Silverlon, are not recognized by the medical community. I hope that, by letting people know about these treatments, and about the phenomena (the dysfunctions, really) that keep these treatments hidden from the public, my readers will lead the way, and that your life—or the life of a loved one—will be saved.

Finding other, similarly lifesaving treatments, turned out to be far easier than I had thought it would be. I didn't have to look very far. A combination of Internet research and "people research" led me to the other three treatments I write about in this book.

Intravenous Alpha Lipoic Acid

Intravenous Alpha Lipoic Acid

As mentioned in Chapter 1, intravenous alpha lipoic acid (IV ALA), also known as thioctic acid, is an intravenous therapy and a naturally occurring compound. Its therapeutic uses include diabetes, atherosclerosis, neurodegenerative disorders, liver diseases, and other conditions. (http://www.epic4health.com/allipacitsro.html)

Pioneered by Dr. Burt Berkson (MD, MS, PhD), intravenous alpha lipoic acid was first used in the 1970s (NIH and Case Western Reserve Affiliated Hospitals) for regenerating organs, especially livers and reversing the complications of diabetes mellitis.

In the next three chapters, you will hear from intravenous alpha lipoic acid pioneer Burt Berkson, and two of his patients, Mary Jo Bean and Paul Marez. In Chapter 4, Dr. Berkson will tell the dramatic story of how he first discovered ALA for the treatment of liver disease, and how his higher-ups at the prestigious medical institution where he was a resident castigated him for using it, even though it miraculously healed his patients. The expressed reason for their anger: He had not followed orders. They had not told him to use ALA. In fact, incredible as it seems, they had specifically told him *not* to do anything to try to save his patients, but rather, to stand by and watch them die.

Luckily for his patients, Dr. Berkson disobeyed their orders.

He will also tell how, years later, in private practice in Las Cruces, New Mexico, he came to use IV ALA in combination with Low Dose Naltrexone (LDN) to successfully treat some very resistant cancers, including Stage IV pancreatic cancer.

Through his story, you will see why so many proponents of integrative medicine consider Dr. Berkson a hero.

In Chapter 5, you'll learn how intravenous ALA cured Mary Jo Bean of her end-stage liver disease (cirrhosis and hepatitis C—a deadly combination), after doctors told her she had from two to twelve months to live, even with the highly toxic pharmaceutical treatments they offered her. She turned their treatments down, and on her own, found Dr. Berkson.

In Chapter 6, you'll learn about how ALA, in combination with LDN, cured Paul Marez of his Stage IV pancreatic cancer—after the doctors at MD Anderson Cancer Center had told him to go home and get his affairs in order. One doctor there even asked Paul if he had considered committing suicide.

Luckily, Mary Jo and Paul decided to look further than their doctors. Both of them are still alive eight years after finding Dr. Berkson. They don't show any signs of dying at the present time. In fact, both are alive and thriving, thanks to ALA and Dr. Berkson.

CHAPTER 4

Burt Berkson, MD, MS, PhD: Pioneer

His Work with IV Alpha Lipoic Acid (ALA) and Oral Low Dose Naltrexone (LDN); His Perceptions About Our Medical System

I first learned about Dr. Burt Berkson's fascinating work with intravenous alpha lipoic acid long before I began thinking about writing this book. It was in 1999, nine years after Tim was first diagnosed with a cancerous brain tumor. Hungry for nutritional solutions for Tim, I started attending meetings of NOHA (Nutrition for Optimal Health Association: http://www.nutrition4health.org), an organization that presented lectures on cutting-edge nutritional treatments.

Dr. Berkson spoke at one of these meetings. His lecture was a paradigm-shifting event for me, because he talked about how, as a resident, he had used a non-traditional treatment that unquestionably saved lives, only to be roundly chastised by his superiors for using it. I found this shocking.

Years later, when my husband's doctors expressed doubts that Silverlon had actually healed Tim's non-healing skin (Chapters 2 and 3), I was reminded of Dr. Berkson's experiences. My husband's doctors reacted very much the way Dr. Berkson's superiors had. Both sets of doctors weren't at all interested in any treatment they themselves weren't "up on." They all showed the same lack of curiosity, and demonstrated an eerily similar hostility toward some really cutting-edge treatments that had saved patients' lives.

In this chapter, Dr. Berkson also tells us how the papers he published on his successes with intravenous alpha lipoic acid garnered interest from the National Institutes of Health (NIH). I want my readers to see that all the treatments I am featuring in this book have a great deal of evidence to back them up, including scholarly papers and studies. Most of these treatments, however, do not have the "gold standard": the randomized double-blind clinical trials that only pharmaceutical companies and the government can afford. (The Ketogenic Diet is the exception. In Section 3, you will learn about the successful Class 1 randomized double-blind trial performed in 2008 by Dr. Helen Cross in the United Kingdom.)

Dr. Berkson includes observations about how the medical system functions, how conventional doctors think, and why it is so difficult for conventional doctors to accept non-standard-of-care treatments like the ones I am profiling in this book. He also points out that large medical institutions often squelch doctors who are creative and curious.

Creativity and curiosity are the cornerstones of the professionals who have pioneered the treatments I am writing about.

Lastly, Dr. Berkson gives us a glimpse into Dr. Bernard Bihari's work with Low Dose Naltrexone. After reading this chapter, I hope you will understand why I consider both Dr. Berkson and Dr. Bihari to be two of my personal heroes.

In Dr. Berkson's words …

I actually started out wanting to be a biology professor, not a medical doctor. I got my MS degree in Biology from Eastern Illinois University, and my PhD from the University of Illinois at Urbana. I wrote my dissertation on the cell biology of microorganisms. I then accepted a professorship at Rutgers, where I both taught and conducted research. I loved it. While I was at Rutgers,

I was on several university medical school committees and slowly developed an interest in clinical medicine.

At this time, my wife Ann began having miscarriages, one after another. She had five of them in all. I had thought that if a person was the head of a department at the University of Chicago or Harvard or Stanford, they really knew more than anybody else. So, we went to doctors like this. And still she'd have these miscarriages in the second trimester, in the fourth to sixth month. These doctors would always say, "These babies are normal. Just get her pregnant again. Maybe next time she'll be able to carry the baby."

In desperation, I went to the medical library, and read some of the journals in obstetrics. This was in the late 1960s. I saw that there was a Dr. Shirodkar in India who said that when people had normal babies with second-trimester miscarriages, it was usual that when they had a D & C on one of the first miscarriages, the cervix was injured or lacerated, so when the baby got to a certain size, the cervix couldn't hold that baby. This 1973 paper in the *Canadian Medical Association Journal* describes Dr. Shirodkar's technique: http://www.pubmedcentral.nih.gov/articlerender.fcgi?artid=1941378.

After completing this research, I went back to Ann's doctor at this prestigious university, and told him about Dr. Shirodkar's procedure. He looked at me and said, "You're a microbiologist. I don't tell you how to practice your field. Don't tell me how to practice gynecology."

"Here's the article. Why don't you read it?" I handed it to him.

"I'm the head of the department. I know what I'm doing. Just get her pregnant again," he said.

So I looked all around the United States for a medical doctor who had studied with Dr. Shirodkar, and found Martin Clyman in New York. Ann became pregnant again, and I took her to Dr. Clyman's office.

He said, "I'll put a little stitch in there—a little ligature, a simple little circular stitch."

Dr. Clyman performed the procedure, and Ann had a normal baby. And then she had another one, five years later.

It was these experiences with Ann's doctors that made me start losing faith in many people in the medical profession. I didn't really want to be a medical doctor, but I thought it might be a good idea for me to have an MD in addition to my PhD. It would help me at the university—it would give me more power there. And I also could be an ombudsman for family members, if they had to deal with medical doctors. That's why I picked up the MD. But I never thought that I would ever stop being a professor.

So I went to medical school. While I was a resident in internal medicine in a teaching hospital in Cleveland, Ohio, I had a very upsetting experience that made me decide to stay in medicine, rather than go back to teaching.

I thought I had been doing well as a resident. But one day the chief of medicine came by and said, "I am very upset with you."

"Why?" I asked. I thought he was kidding.

"You have no deaths on your service. Most people have seen several deaths by now and you haven't seen any," he replied.

I told him that I really try to keep people alive.

"It's very unusual. I'm going to give you two people who will surely die," he said. "They have acute and fulminant liver disease. They ate poisonous mushrooms, and the expert on liver disease said we cannot get a transplant for them, and nothing can save them. So I want you to go upstairs, watch them die, take notes and present this to grand medical rounds." In addition, he told me that the patients were my responsibility.

I went upstairs. I looked at these two very sick people. And as a medical doctor, especially in internal medicine, you're supposed to follow the orders of the chief, just like a private in the army would follow the orders of a sergeant. But I had six years of education above my medical training, for a master's and a PhD in microbiology and cell biology, and I was always looking for new things. So I called Washington and spoke to the head of the National Institutes of Health in Internal Medicine, Dr. Fred Bartter. I asked him, "Is there anything in the world that you know of that might regenerate a liver?"

Dr. Bartter said he was studying intravenous alpha lipoic acid because he knew it would reverse diabetic neuropathy and other complications of diabetes. When he gave it to people, ALA seemed to regenerate their organs, stimulating their stem cells to start growing and to regenerate new organ tissue.

He sent me the alpha lipoic acid. I picked it up at the Cleveland airport about three hours later. The commercial pilot handed it to me. I ran back to the hospital and injected it into these two people for a period of two weeks. After two weeks, their livers had regenerated fully. And they're still alive and well today, in their eighties, some thirty years later.

I was very excited. The people at NIH were very interested in my patients. But the medical chiefs of the hospital were not happy with me. In fact, they seemed angry.

They said, "We told the families that these people were going to die, that there was no hope. And now they're alive and well. You know, it makes us look bad. And you did something without asking us for permission."

I said, "You told me that these people were my responsibility, so I did what I thought was correct."

I asked them if they wanted to know what it was that I gave my patients.

They said, "No." They didn't want to know. They were not even curious. They said, "This is not an approved drug. It's not on our formulary. And you did not follow orders like a good internal medicine doctor."

I was sort of discouraged by this. It was very different from what I had seen as a professor of biology. Whenever I discovered something new in biology, everybody would pat me on the back and give me awards. In medicine, it seemed to me that if you discovered something new, you were thought of as an outlaw.

When more people who had eaten poisonous mushrooms came into the hospital, I was told I should not give them whatever it was I had given the first patients. Poisonous mushrooms destroy the liver. There's not much you can do for these folks, except a transplant or, in this case, alpha lipoic acid. I gave these patients alpha lipoic acid anyway, and they got better, too.

The National Institutes of Health started supporting my work. I think because of this, the people at the hospital I was at had to go along with what I was doing. Eventually Dr. Bartter and I published a paper on seventy-nine people with so-called terminal liver disease, describing how seventy-five of these patients regenerated their livers, with just intravenous lipoic acid. Our paper was published in 1980 as part of the proceedings of the 1978 International Amanita Symposium in Heidelberg, Germany. (http://honest medicine.typepad.com/BERKSON-1980-amanitin.pdf) And my first short note about this was in the *New England Journal of Medicine*. (http://www.ncbi.nlm.nih.gov/pubmed/366411?ordinalpos=3&itool=EntrezSystem2.PEntrez.Pubmed.Pubmed_ResultsPanel.Pubmed_DefaultReportPanel.Pubmed_RVDocSum)

The NIH was very excited about our work, and was interested in conducting a big study on ALA. However, their interest waned when, sadly, Dr. Bartter passed away in the early 1980s. But even before his death, no large pharmaceutical company was interested in sponsoring our work, possibly because they would have had to pay too much money to the Germans for the ability to use their patent. (The Germans already had a patent on ALA.)

Personally, I also believe that because ALA is effective for many different diseases, no pharmaceutical company wants to go through the expensive clinical trial approval process. In order to make the most money, they want one medication per disease. For example, if a pharmaceutical company were to get ALA approved for liver disease, they would lose money on their diabetes mellitus drug, because ALA is also effective for reversing the complications of diabetes. And because no pharmaceutical company would be sponsoring our work, there would be no one taking out ads in the medical journals, or doctors and hospitals buying reprints from them. Medical journals rely on ads and reprints for a large portion of their income. So this was a losing proposition all the way around. In other words, alpha lipoic acid could save lives, but because it was such an inexpensive substance and a natural product, it would not make anyone a significant amount of money.

Even so, there was some interest in my work. Dr. Bartter and I were invited to Europe to be visiting scientists at the Max Planck Institute for a conference on liver disease and mushroom poisoning. I also kept having more and more successes in Cleveland. As I said, the chiefs had to put up with me. After we had four patients with such remarkable results, Dr. Bartter and several other doctors flew into Cleveland and set up a national conference on organ regeneration. I was the lead speaker. I don't think the older doctors liked that very much.

For twenty-three years, I was the principal FDA investigator for the intravenous use of alpha lipoic acid. I'm also the expert consultant to the Centers for Disease Control on alpha lipoic acid and liver poisoning.

Pharmaceutical companies, though, weren't interested in doing more investigation. It might surprise you to know that I'm not criticizing the pharmaceutical companies. I think this is just business to them, and here in America, medicine is a business. It's just the way things are done. If somebody wants to get a drug approved by the FDA, they have to spend hundreds of millions of dollars to do it. Even if the research has already been done in prestigious hospitals in Asia or in Europe, they still have to do the research all over again in the United States. And if the Germans own a drug's patent, an American company may not get full control of that patent. So most pharmaceutical companies are not willing to spend all that money to get alpha lipoic acid approved by the FDA. Would you? I mean, if you were a multi-millionaire, would you spend all this money to get a drug approved, if others could undersell your product? You would lose your multi-million-dollar investment!

The problem here is that no one has found a way to make big money on intravenous alpha lipoic acid. So, even though it is efficacious, it's a losing endeavor for any corporation to promote it.

People often ask me why more doctors have not come out in favor of my work with alpha lipoic acid, or in favor of any of the other treatments this book covers, for that matter. I can only point to the way doctors are educated. In fact, it's a misnomer to say they are educated at all. Most of their work is training, rather than education.

In medicine, they talk about training. In biology, we talk about education. There is a big difference. When I started medical school in Chicago many, many years ago, I used to ask questions. The anatomy professor took me aside and said, "You know, we give you information and you memorize it and give it back to us. And if you do this, and you pass the test, in four years, you're a medical doctor. We tell you what to do, and you do things just like we do it." And he added, "If you don't do it our way, you will have to do the year over again."

This was very different from the way I was educated for my PhD. There, we were encouraged to ask questions and to think creatively. In other words, we were educated, not trained. But in medical school, it's training; it's technical. It's not like a biological education. It's a very different type of educational process. Medicine is training, and if people are trained, they'll all do the same thing in the same way all of the time.

Even when a patient comes to me, and it's obvious that their hepatitis C, for instance, is in total remission after my treatments, it isn't surprising to me that when they go back to their original doctor, he or she will not believe that the intravenous alpha lipoic acid has helped. They simply can't accept that a treatment they think they didn't learn about in medical school, or from their medical journals, is having such positive results, when their own treatments have failed. Ironically, they all learn about alpha lipoic acid in medical school. However, most doctors forget about it.

Frankly, it doesn't help the situation that pharmaceutical companies—which control the clinical trials that are conducted on their own drugs, as well as the articles that are published in the medical journals—also have a tremendous influence on what appears on the media. For instance, in 2007, I was invited by the National Cancer Institute to fly to Washington and give them a lecture on how I was using alpha lipoic acid, combined with Low Dose Naltrexone, to treat autoimmune disease and cancer. I was very surprised that it was so well received.

At the same meeting, Dr. Maira Gironi flew in from Italy, and spoke about how she was having magnificent results reversing MS with just a little bit of Low Dose Naltrexone at bedtime. In April 2008, Dr. Gironi presented a paper on this study at the 60th annual meeting of the American Academy of Neurology in Chicago. (http://honestmedicine.typepad.com/Gironi-AAN-T-Apr-15-LDN. pdf. Go to Course Number P02.149 on p. 38—actual page 4 of this document.) However, I understand that her successes with LDN were not publicized in the press. Instead, another—more expensive—drug for MS, manufactured by a large pharmaceutical company, received a tremendous amount of press coverage. Here is the press release, put out by Novartis, about this other drug: http://honestmedicine.typepad.com/NOVARTIS-RELEASE-COMI_249738.pdf. It's a shame.

But I can't let all this get me down.

In more recent years, some of the most interesting work I've done, and had great results with, has been with a combination of alpha lipoic acid and Low Dose Naltrexone. The way I found Low Dose Naltrexone is really very interesting. One day, thirteen years ago, a man came into my office with a walker. He could hardly move. He was about 70 years old. I asked him what was wrong, and he told me that he had just been to MD Anderson Cancer Center, and they told him he had prostate cancer, metastasized to his bones. He also had lupus and rheumatoid arthritis. They told him he only had a few months to live. Nothing could be done.

"Why are you in *my* office?" I asked him.

He said he had a wife with dementia and a son with a mental disability. He had to have them placed in a nursing home before he died. I asked what I could do for him. He said he really needed some narcotics to handle the pain. I said I'd be glad to write that prescription for him.

Then he asked me if I'd ever heard of Dr. Bernard Bihari in New York. I said, "No, I never heard of him." He told me that he had heard that Dr. Bihari was curing cancer.

I said, "I don't know why you're in my office, or MD Anderson, or the Mayo Clinic. I don't see any great results for curing cancer from any of these places. I don't know how to cure cancer. So why don't you go up and see him?"

"Well, he's just in a little office in New York. What does he know?" he said.

I told him the story of when I was at a university hospital with alpha lipoic acid, which was really effective at regenerating livers and many other organs, too, and they just didn't want to hear about it. They were in the liver transplant business. I added, "Maybe if this Dr. Bihari was at a big medical center like Sloan-Kettering or MD Anderson, and he had discovered a simple cure for cancer, they would have probably thrown him out, because such a discovery would put them out of business."

What I said must have convinced him, because he went and saw Dr. Bihari.

And I didn't see him for three years.

Three years later, he walked in without his walker, a normal guy.

I said, "John, how are you doing?"

"You know, the wind's blowing. My nose is stuffed. I really need something for these allergies," he said.

"But, John, what about the cancer?"

"Oh, Dr. Bihari cured that," he said in a very relaxed way.

"What about the lupus and rheumatoid arthritis?"

"Oh, he cured that, too."

I asked, "What did he use?"

"Did you ever hear of naltrexone?"

I said, "Sure, it's something doctors administer to heroin addicts because it occupies their opiate receptors. When they shoot up, they don't feel the heroin."

"Well, Dr. Bihari found that if you take a tiny amount of naltrexone, a very low dose, at bedtime, it fools the brain into thinking there aren't enough natural opiates in the bloodstream," John said. "Then, in the early hours of the morning, large amounts of natural opiates are released from the brain and from the rest of the nervous system to modulate the immune system to fight cancer and to help autoimmune disease."

This explanation made sense to me, but I was still very skeptical. My interest was piqued, though, because my wife had two aunts who had lupus and rheumatoid arthritis. They were actually on chemotherapy drugs, like methotrexate, and steroids, like prednisone, that swelled them up. The methotrexate was killing their bone marrow and damaging their hearts. They weren't getting any better. So, I asked them if they wanted to try this Low Dose Naltrexone. They said, "Sure." In one month, they were completely normal, off all drugs, and only taking this $12 a month prescription.

I had around one hundred patients who were suffering with lupus, rheumatoid arthritis, dermatomyositis and other autoimmune diseases. I would say that within one month, 85 percent of them were off all medications and feeling normal. As I started treating more and more people with autoimmune diseases, I began using LDN in combination with intravenous ALA—with excellent results. In fact, I believe that in most cases, my results with the combination treatment for autoimmune diseases are even better than results with LDN or ALA alone.

I've also had some wonderful successes treating cancers, including pancreatic cancers, with a combination of these two drugs. One of my patients came to me after being told by MD Anderson that he would die within a few months. He had pancreatic cancer, and so had nothing to lose. He was eager to try alpha lipoic acid and Low Dose Naltrexone in combination. He has since been alive and active, and still working, for eight years. (Editor's note: Dr. Berkson is referring here to Paul Marez, who tells his story in Chapter 6.)

It is quite incredible, because pancreatic cancer is one of the cancers considered a death sentence by oncologists. They're pretty much in agreement on that. In 2006, I published my results, a case study, in *Integrative Cancer Therapies*. (http://www.ldn4cancer.

com/files/Berkson_Pancreatic_paper.pdf) In 2009, the same publication published another paper on three more successes with this deadly disease. The abstract is here: http://ict.sagepub.com/cgi/content/abstract/8/4/416. And on April 25, 2009, I gave an invitational lecture at the first European LDN Conference at Glasgow University, Scotland. The Europeans are very interested in this therapy because it costs so much less than the conventional approach.

I don't think I can tell you how wonderful it is to be able to help patients who have life-threatening conditions, such as hepatitis, lupus, MS, cancer and a whole host of other ailments. The pharmaceutical treatments these patients' doctors offer them aren't working well, so their doctors just give up on them. I hope that, as more and more patients have success with treatments like the ones featured in this book, they will wake up, start doing their own research, and find treatments on their own.

But still, I would never force anybody to try any of the treatments I use. I ask them, "What do you want to do? Do you want to stick with the rheumatologist?" (Actually, I tell them always to stick with their rheumatologist or their oncologist.) "Or do you want to try something a little different?"

Many of them say, "No, I'm really happy with what I'm doing."

And I say, "That's fine." I would never want to force anything on anyone, and I don't want anybody to force anything on me. People should be free to use any reasonable medical treatment protocol they think will help them.

The first people with mushroom poisoning Dr. Berkson treated over thirty years ago, Eunice and John Goostree, still stay in touch with him. They remain two of his biggest fans. In fact, Eunice Goostree wrote a review on Amazon.com of Dr. Berkson's book, *The Alpha Lipoic Acid Breakthrough*. You may read her review here: http://www.amazon.com/Alpha-Lipoic-Acid-Breakthrough-Antioxidant/dp/0761514570.

Over the years, in Las Cruces, Dr. Berkson has saved many patients from needing liver transplants. He suspects that the fact that he has saved them from needing liver transplants may be one reason the medical establishment is not enthusiastic about his use of intravenous alpha lipoic acid. Transplants, he pointed out to me in a recent phone conversation, are a huge business in many US hospitals.

Patients come to Dr. Berkson from all over the world, and he has a waiting list of nearly a year. Luckily for Mary Jo Bean and Paul Marez—as shared in the next two chapters—and thousands of other patients who have been cured by Dr. Berkson in the last twenty-five years, Dr. Berkson opted to leave institutional medicine. We are grateful to him!

If you enjoyed this chapter, I hope you'll want to listen to my interview with Dr. Berkson on HonestMedicine.com at http://www.honestmedicine.com/2009/02/audio-interview-burt-berkson-md-phd-talks-with-honest-medicine-about-his-work-with-alpha-lipoic-acid.html. You can also find a link to the word-for-word transcription of this interview by scrolling down on the web page.

CHAPTER 5

Mary Jo Bean

Hepatitis C and Cirrhosis of the Liver:
Intravenous Alpha Lipoic Acid

Like the other patient advocates featured in this book, Mary Jo Bean and I have become good friends. Like me, and like the other advocates, she is extremely committed to getting her message out to the world. She believes that once a person's health has been turned around by a treatment like intravenous ALA— a treatment that the medical establishment doesn't know about, doesn't want to know about, and doesn't recommend—or if you've had a loved one who's had this experience, you've got to do your part to tell everyone who will listen.

Like all the other patient advocates who tell their stories in this book, Mary Jo had to find the patient-evidence-based treatment that saved her life on her own.

Her story is an inspiration.

In May 2002, when I was 66 years old, I was diagnosed with chronic hepatitis C and severe cirrhosis of the liver. Exploratory surgery showed that my liver was very badly damaged: hard as a rock, and with only one small part of the left lobe functioning. Doctors said it was so bad that I must have had liver disease for at least twenty-five years.

I was never a drinker, so the doctors believed that, most probably, I had contracted the cirrhosis from blood transfusions. Between 1956 and 1970, before blood was checked for the virus, I had had many surgeries where I needed blood: a tubal ligation in 1959, a partial hysterectomy in 1962, and a complete hysterectomy in 1964. And in 1970, I had surgery to have a cyst removed. The surgeons got too close to a main artery, and I hemorrhaged really, really badly, and almost died. In every instance, they gave me blood. Most people today don't know this, but back then, any wino could walk into a blood bank and donate a pint of blood and walk out with five bucks in his hand. And they'd do the same thing the next month, and the next; and they were never, ever tested for hepatitis.

But while I knew where I had probably gotten the cirrhosis, I only knew how I did *not* get the hepatitis: I did not get it from using drugs or engaging in illicit sex. I never did either.

But how I got the liver disease isn't the important thing. It's the treatment that's important. When the doctors told me that I only had two months to a year to live, they said that the only way I would even live a year was if I went on the drug Interferon. I didn't know one thing about Interferon or about cirrhosis.

I decided that if I was going to die of this disease, I'd find out everything I could about it and about the treatment the doctors were recommending for me. So, I went to a support group in Oklahoma City at Baptist Hospital. I talked to many patients who were either on Interferon or had been on it, and they told me it was mostly ineffective, and that—just as bad—it had horrible side effects. There were big, strapping men there and they not only were very ill on the drug, they also told me they had contemplated suicide on it, to the point that a family member had to stay with them around the clock. The drug caused horrible depression. I knew that if they were feeling bad on it, I wouldn't be able to stand it, since I'd always been a really skinny gal.

To me, the scariest thing was that even the doctors admitted that Interferon was a difficult drug when they said that a family member would have to stay with me around the clock while I was being infused with it. I had a husband, a daughter, and three adopted boys, and I just didn't want to put them through all of that. I decided that, even though I loved my family and my life, I'd rather be dead than live this way.

To me the choice wasn't hard at all. I went out and planned my funeral, paid for my cremation, bought my headstone, and gave a bunch of my things away. I said, "I've had a good life. I'm getting ready to die." I made all the plans to die, and no plans to live; I was that sure.

But still, even though I had made my decision, the doctors kept pushing me to have the Interferon. Sometimes I think it was the money factor, although I can't be sure, and I hate to think that way. But they really pushed it. Even after I had decided I wouldn't do it, my doctor had his physician's assistant call me to tell me that I would die if I didn't come into the office right away to start on the Interferon. I was so mad that I went to his office and told my doctor again, to his face, that there was no way I would take the drug. I even said that there was no way I was going to go on "that crap."

He insisted, "You need to be on it."

I said, "It's my money, my body, my life, my choice. I'm not doing it."

He just walked out of the room.

I did not know what I was going to do, but I knew for sure that I did not want to take Interferon. I began praying and asking God to give me the wisdom to know what to do. Finally, I made a decision to try to find a natural treatment. I had never had any dealings with any natural treatments or holistic doctors, but somehow, I just knew that I should go that route.

But finding such a doctor, especially in rural Oklahoma where I live, didn't come overnight, or without problems. I discovered Dr. Berkson's treatment in a most unusual way. One day, I was lying on the couch, so sick I couldn't even get up. I couldn't do anything, even clean my house, so the clutter had just piled up. I was feeling so worthless. I asked my husband to hand me the junk mail and the trash can, thinking, "Maybe I can at least go through the junk mail and feel like I am worth something." I think I was also secretly hoping I'd find something about liver disease there. I know that sounds crazy, but I also know that God planted that thought; I just know it. The first thing I picked up from the pile of junk mail wasn't anything. But the second piece of mail was a flyer from the Whitaker Wellness Institute, a holistic treatment center in Newport Beach, California. I wasn't even on Dr. Whitaker's mailing list; I had never seen his newsletter. In fact, I had never, ever gotten anything from them before, and at that time, I certainly wasn't into holistic medicine, although I sure am now! But I knew that some way, somehow, God was going to show me what to do.

I read the flyer. It was an article about Dr. Burt Berkson in Las Cruces, New Mexico. It told about how he was curing people with liver disease with a treatment called intravenous alpha lipoic acid. After I read the article, I went out and got Dr. Berkson's book, *The Alpha Lipoic Acid Breakthrough*. I read it twice. I knew then, without a doubt, that this was the treatment I needed to take, that this was what I was supposed to do.

When I first called Dr. Berkson's office, I just asked lots of questions; I didn't even give them my name. I waited about two days and I called back and made an appointment. This was the first week in November 2002, and they couldn't see me until December. By December 10, I was so sick. I weighed around eighty-two pounds, and could barely talk above a whisper. And I couldn't walk without assistance. The clinic was about 700 miles away from where I live. At about seventy miles from home, I started crying. I was in so much pain. I begged my husband, "Just turn around and go back home, so I can die." I told him that I'd never make it to Las Cruces.

My husband told me to shut up, and this time, I listened to him. He said, "I'm not stopping until we get to Las Cruces. This is the last hope we've got."

We made it to Las Cruces. At that time, Dr. Berkson's clinic was really small, a hole in the wall, behind a tiny Italian restaurant. I said, "What on God's green earth have we got ourselves into?" The whole office was so small you couldn't even turn around. The nurse would be giving you an IV treatment and her backside would be sticking in somebody else's face. The room was that small!

We met Dr. Berkson, and he started asking me questions. I told him that the doctors had told me that I had two to twelve months to live. And that had been seven months previous. He looked at me, and he reached across the little table (he didn't even have a desk then), and he put his hand on mine, and said, "Mrs. Bean, only God knows when you're going to die."

You know, those other doctors had stripped me of every inch, every hair of hope that I had. But what Dr. Berkson said in those few words gave me hope. When you take somebody's hope from them, you might as well just slit their throat, because you have to have hope. And after all I've been through, I have to say that I don't believe that there is any such thing as "false hope."

Dr. Berkson asked me if I wanted to start treatment that day and I said, "Yes, that is why I am here." So I took my first treatment that day. I went back to the motel and slept like a baby, something I had not done in two years or more. The next morning, I had to go to the lab and get more tests, then back to the clinic for another treatment and a visit with Dr. Berkson. On that second visit to him, I told him that I would like to get another opinion. What made me say that, I will never know. I never even thought I wanted a second opinion before I heard myself say it. But Dr. Berkson was fine with that, and he sent me to another doctor in Las Cruces, a Dr. Prasad Podila, a highly respected gastroenterologist. He got me an appointment for seven o'clock the next morning. I had never heard of such a thing. I went in, and Dr. Podila looked at all my records, and asked me some questions. Then he got right up close to me and shook his finger in my face, and he said, "Mrs. Bean, I have watched Dr. Berkson for years. I've seen patients before and after he's treated them. You are very, very wise to be going to Dr. Berkson."

Dr. Podila told me three times that morning that I was very, very wise to be going to Dr. Berkson. There isn't a doubt in my mind that the reason I asked for another opinion and the reason that Dr. Podila told me three times that I was wise to be going to Dr. Berkson was so that I would know, without a doubt, that my going to Dr. Berkson was an answer to my prayer for wisdom, and was definitely from God.

Dr. Berkson continued my treatments that day. I stayed two weeks, taking ten treatments, as well as going on the diet, and starting the vitamins and nutritional supplements he told me to take. (Editor's note: The nutrient-rich diet and nutritional supplements Dr. Berkson prescribes are listed in the Appendix.) Each day I felt stronger.

In fact, after the third treatment I wanted to go to Walmart to shop! When I arrived home, I unpacked all by myself and did all the laundry. The next morning I got up and cleaned our 2,000-square-foot home, dusting, mopping, vacuuming, and even cleaning the ceiling fans by myself. These were all things I had not been able to do in over a year. But now, I had so much energy.

I went back to Las Cruces to the clinic again two months later, but this time my husband didn't have to go with me. I drove a friend who was very ill, and needed to see Dr. Berkson. I did all the driving, the loading and unloading of the car and taking care of my friend for two weeks while each of us took ten treatments. My labs were improving, but the greatest thing was my increased energy. After all this time, everything was completely turning around for me.

For the next year and a half, I went to Las Cruces for five treatments every three to four months. Then I began to stretch it out longer, once waiting seven months before going for five treatments—one per day.

Only four months after starting the IV alpha lipoic acid treatments, an MRI and blood tests showed that my liver was almost totally rebuilt. After six months of treatments, I power-washed our entire house, and painted all the outside trim with two coats. I put in a fair-sized garden by myself, and put the veggies in the freezer. And just as amazing, I made two trips of 1,200 miles each by myself. And every month and every year since, I have stayed healthy.

My Oklahoma doctors have been kind of strange about my success with Dr. Berkson's treatments. The doctor who told me I only had two to twelve months to live seemed interested at first, even impressed. But after a while, he showed no more interest at all in my progress.

I am so thankful that God not only showed me that Interferon was not for me, but also led me to Dr. Berkson, who was able to return me to health. He and his staff treat the whole person—body, mind and spirit. After just one visit with Dr. Berkson, I had hope, and each day that hope grew. I felt a genuine caring about me as a patient and as a person, a rare thing these days in the medical community. In his book, *The Alpha Lipoic Acid Breakthrough*, Dr. Berkson says that he tries to put himself in every patient's shoes, and I truly believe that he does. I have watched him with patients for over seven years now, and I have never seen or heard anything but wonderful things about him. My friends and family all see me now and say that I am a miracle. I owe it all first to God, then to Dr. Berkson for his wisdom and his caring.

As a bonus to the wonderful treatment I've received at the Berkson Clinic, I have met some of the most wonderful friends, other patients who are also seeing their lives turn around. At first, I met patients mainly with terminal liver disease, but now, I am also meeting patients with other diseases, including cancer. They are having great results, too. But just as wonderful, there are no long, sad faces there. Even though everyone is fighting destructive diseases, we have hope and everyone wears a smile. We are survivors.

In February 2006, I started a support group for the hepatitis patients who go to Dr. Berkson. The group has grown to include over four hundred people, several with other diseases, too. I have had people from all over the world call or email me about Dr. Berkson. It has been the most rewarding thing I have ever done, and every time I reach out to someone with encouragement and help, it comes back to me tenfold. It has given me more happiness than I could have ever imagined.

I feel like the most blessed woman alive. In 2005 and again in February 2007, I had CAT scans and ultrasounds, as well as extensive lab work done, and all showed that my liver was completely rebuilt and there was no sign of the cirrhosis. The hepatitis virus is still there but it is under control and I have no problem with it. I continue to go to the clinic for alpha lipoic acid treatments twice a year and I stay on the diet and the vitamin and supplement regimen. My scans and lab work remain excellent, as does my energy.

Word has gotten around about Dr. Berkson. People come to the clinic from all over the country, and all over the world. Now it takes six to eight months to get an appointment. So, if I find someone who is even vaguely contemplating going to him, I tell them to make the appointment now!

I cannot end this chapter without adding that Dr. Berkson's staff is the greatest staff I have ever seen anywhere. His wife, Ann, heads up the office. She is a wonderful lady, and so helpful. Everyone loves her. Dee, Mary Kay and Rebecca (the Berksons' daughter-in-law) also work in the office and are so sweet. Then, there is Linda, the head nurse, technician and Dr. Berkson's right hand. She is a real Florence Nightingale. I haven't met one patient who doesn't love Linda. Sue is Linda's right hand and assistant and is following right in Linda's footsteps. She is a wonderful lady, too. No one can walk into that clinic without feeling genuine caring for their well-being.

I have written this chapter as my way of thanking God and Dr. Berkson, and to try in some way to help others with liver diseases, and other so-called "terminal" illnesses, to know that there is a way to good health without filling their bodies full of drugs that kill healthy cells and destroy immune systems.

Mary Jo is now 74 years old. Her husband, Lavan, has many health issues that take up a great deal of her time and energy. Yet, she still works tirelessly to get the word out about Dr. Berkson. Mary Jo has accompanied many of her friends to Las Cruces to see Dr. Berkson, and now has close friendships with hundreds of his patients, making herself available by phone to anyone who wants to talk with her. She answers their questions from the patient perspective. At first, only hepatitis and cirrhosis patients were contacting her. But soon, people with cancer, lupus, Parkinson's, MS, scleroderma, fibromyalgia, Lyme disease, and many other autoimmune diseases began to contact her, as well. She started out by doing research for them and sending them information about Dr. Berkson's treatment for their particular disease(s). She keeps in touch several times a week with her email list of four hundred. Mary Jo feels that this is the least she can do. "Dr. Berkson gave me my life back," she says. "I want the world to know about him."

CHAPTER 6

Paul Marez

Stage IV Pancreatic Cancer, Metastasized to the Liver:
Intravenous Alpha Lipoic Acid and Oral LDN

Before Paul Marez learned that he had pancreatic cancer with metastases to the liver (and only four months to live), he didn't even know what an oncologist was. He was to soon find out. Paul's story is so inspiring because, in some way, I believe it was a combination of his lack of knowledge of things medical, and his skeptical nature that gave him the courage to question the so-called wisdom of the "big shots" at a major teaching hospital, and to think outside the box.

I first learned about Paul from Dr. Berkson, who wrote about Paul's story in a case study that was published in *Integrative Cancer Therapies,* a peer-reviewed journal. (http://ict.sagepub.com/cgi/content/short/5/1/83) I told Dr. Berkson that I really wanted Paul's story to be part of this book. After all, pancreatic cancer, especially Stage IV pancreatic cancer, is one of the most "hopeless." And conventional medicine has had very little success with it. Dr. Berkson, on the other hand, has had some really impressive results.

Dr. Berkson worried about asking Paul to participate, because Paul is a very private person. Still, I wanted to include Paul's story. So, I spoke with Mary Jo, who had already agreed to be part of the book, and she contacted Paul for me. He agreed to participate.

I am so glad Paul overcame his quiet nature to help me to educate people about Dr. Berkson. There are so many people in situations like Paul's, who listen to their conventional doctors, and undergo conventional treatments, very often with negative outcomes. I hope they will read Paul's story and feel encouraged to seek out treatments, like intravenous alpha lipoic acid, and the other patient-evidence-based treatments featured in this book.

In Paul's words …

I am really glad to be a part of any project that lets the public know about Dr. Berkson. I tell anyone who will listen about him all the time. Getting a diagnosis, like I did, of pancreatic cancer that has metastasized to the liver, is devastating. Dr. Berkson was the first doctor who said he could help me. And, more importantly, he did.

Back in 2002, I was having bad stomach pains. I went to a doctor in our local hospital in Alamogordo, which is about fifteen miles from where I live in Cloudcroft, New Mexico. Cloudcroft is a small mountain resort community with only 700 full-time residents, but for some reason, there are lots of people with cancer here. When the first doctor I went to said he was sending me to an oncologist, I didn't even know what that meant. I was kind of naïve back then. After having a biopsy, the oncologist told me I had pancreatic cancer. I was so naïve that I said, "OK, then cut it out."

He said, "It's not quite that easy. What you have can't be treated." And it kind of went downhill from there.

I went on the Internet, and found that people with pancreatic cancer usually live only four to six months. If the doctors hadn't scared me enough, that certainly did. At the time, I was 44 years old, and my wife Becky and I had a 6-year-old son. He's 12 now.

Then I read a *Time* magazine article that said that MD Anderson was one of the best cancer places in the world, so I decided that, if anyone could cure me, it was MD Anderson. I made an appointment there, and Becky and I made reservations to stay a week. (MD Anderson has so many patients coming to them from all over the world that they even have a four-star hotel connected to the hospital. I sometimes call it a "Cancer Walmart.")

But the news was just as depressing at MD Anderson. I had an appointment with two doctors. They said there was nothing they could do, either—that they couldn't help me. They were very blunt, and very to the point. They put a time limit on me, too. "You'll probably live about four months." Just like that.

I told them, "I've made reservations for a week here."

They said, "We've looked at all your records, and we don't see any hope for you." When I showed my obvious disappointment, they really drove the point home. "We can treat you, if you want to die here. Or you can die at home." This is pretty much verbatim. Becky was in tears.

When I asked how they would treat me, if I decided to stay, they said they would put me in a clinical trial. I'd be one of their "test subjects," but they couldn't even promise that I'd get the real medicine. "We have a clinical trial and some patients really get the medicine, and others get sugar pills, and you won't know which you are getting. You may be getting medicine and you may be in the control."

To their credit, I guess, I really didn't encourage me to enter one of their clinical trials. They obviously didn't think anything they had would help me. They said, "You can stay here, and run up a big medical bill, and die. Or you can go home and die, and not run up a big bill." They just came out and flat told me this. One was an oncologist and the other was a student, and they were cold serious. The younger doctor even looked at me and asked, "Have you thought about suicide?" To this day, I am not sure if he was recommending that I try suicide, or if he was testing me psychologically to see if I had thought about ending my life.

I looked at him, and said, "No, I haven't thought about suicide." I was more mad than anything else. So I said, "I think I'll go home."

They said, "That's probably the best choice for you."

And so my wife and I went home, very discouraged. We didn't know what to do. Before we found Dr. Berkson, I think we had tried around five doctors: my oncologist in Alamogordo, the two doctors at MD Anderson and a couple of general family doctors. All of them said the same thing: "There's nothing we can do for you."

But I really wanted to be treated, so an oncologist in Almagordo gave me around fifteen chemotherapy treatments: gemcitabine and carboplatin. There was lots of waiting between treatments because my blood counts were too low. But, the chemo didn't seem to be working anyway. I just kept feeling worse and worse. I began to think of chemotherapy like shoving a shotgun in my stomach and pulling the trigger, hoping that some of the stuff it kills is bad.

Then, Becky, who works for the Cloudcroft school system, found out about Dr. Berkson. One of the teachers was going to him, and encouraged us to go, too. She told Becky that, if anyone could help me, it was Dr. Berkson.

Lots of people were starting to learn about Dr. Berkson, so it was very hard to get in; it's even harder now. But I called him up, and told him how serious my condition was, and how every doctor I had been to had discouraged me. I begged him to see me, and he did. So Becky and I drove to Las Cruces. I brought all my records and x-rays. Dr. Berkson looked everything over very carefully, and talked with me for a long time, a few hours, even though there was a waiting room full of patients. Finally, he said, "I think I may be able to help you. I've had some success with this." I couldn't believe it. I was so happy. He was the first doctor that had told me that.

I said, "You're my doctor! Everyone else I've talked to said they can't do anything for me. Tell me when and how. I'm here." I started the treatments right away, that day: intravenous alpha lipoic acid, a special diet, and vitamins. (Editor's note: The nutrient-rich diet and nutritional supplements Dr. Berkson prescribes are in the Appendix.) And every night, I took 4.5 mg of Low Dose Naltrexone.

Whenever I go to Las Cruces, I listen to the other patients talk. The main topic of conversation usually is, "How did you find this place?" I've been there so many times now, and have sat next to people from New York, Alaska, Hawaii—from all over. Lots of people found Dr. Berkson on the Internet, by searching for treatments for liver disease. Now he's also beginning to show up online when people search for treatments for autoimmune diseases and cancer, too.

I'm blessed, because Cloudcroft is only eighty miles from Las Cruces, so I am able to drive back and forth on a regular basis, and be there in an hour and a half. For a while, I had just one treatment a day. I varied it, and still do, depending on how I've been feeling and how my lab reports and scans look.

I've been able to keep working throughout my treatments—even the chemo—although I did take a lot of sick leave and vacation time. I work for an electric utility company, and have worked there forever. Our company is an electric cooperative; we're like a small family, so whenever I got sick, other people gave me a bunch of their vacation time. Altogether, they gave me 400-500 hours. Even when I was doing the chemo, I would time it so that I'd take off a Friday morning or afternoon, and by Monday, I could be back to work.

But Dr. Berkson's treatments are different. While the chemotherapy made me feel sicker and sicker, with the alpha lipoic acid, I started to feel a lot more energetic right away. Most of the patients I meet in Dr. Berkson's office have the same reaction to ALA. I also follow the diet Dr. Berkson recommends, and take a truckload of vitamins, forty or fifty a day, which he prescribes. The brands he recommends—he sells them there, but we can buy them elsewhere—are very high quality. Most of these brands can only be bought by doctors, and not by the general public.

This treatment has been so effective for me, much more effective than the chemotherapy I took earlier on. I think it's shameful that insurance will pay for chemo, but not for alpha lipoic acid, Low Dose Naltrexone and the supplements Dr. Berkson recommends.

I also find it very disappointing that most other doctors are not at all curious about Dr. Berkson's treatments, even after they see how well I'm doing. And remember, I was considered "terminal." For instance, for a short while, I was doing chemotherapy and alpha lipoic acid at the same time. My oncologist's only response when he learned that I was also being treated with alpha lipoic acid was that, if it wasn't hurting me, he "didn't have a problem" with it. He said, "If it makes you feel better or calms you, that's fine." But he was not at all curious about exactly *what* Dr. Berkson was treating me with.

It's the same way with other doctors who have seen me since my diagnosis. They obviously have to see that I've gotten better with Dr. Berkson's treatment, but they aren't curious, either. Those that notice that I'm still alive, and even thriving, say that I must have been misdiagnosed initially, because "people just don't live with pancreatic cancer."

I think that most conventional doctors, especially oncologists, have blinders on. They only see one vision straight ahead. So, if you can't be treated with chemo or radiation, they figure you're going to die. And if you're not dead without their treatments, you must have been misdiagnosed. That's all they've got, and that's all they're going to give you. And if that doesn't work, well then, nothing can.

Dr. Berkson has helped a lot of people. I have sat there in his office and seen people come in, in very bad shape, like I used to be.

I've seen them come in in wheelchairs, and with oxygen tanks. And within months, I see them up and walking around. One man from Indiana came in, in such bad shape. And he told me he needed a liver transplant, but that his doctors had told him that there was no way he would ever get one, because he used to smoke, and because he was old and overweight. But he read about Dr. Berkson on the Internet, and he said to himself, "What have I got to lose?"

That's pretty much everyone's attitude when they go there. Most of them have been given a death sentence by their doctors. And most of them keep coming back, and every time I see them, they're doing better. This one older guy I mentioned before is doing fine now. He comes in, sits down, and talks to me, and the first time I saw him he was in a wheelchair and on oxygen. The difference is just amazing.

These patients often have funny stories, too. Like that guy. He told me, "I went back and talked to my doctor, the one who told me I'd never get a transplant because I was in such bad shape, that there was no hope for me. I told him, 'Look at me. I'm better.' But the doctor told me he was sure I was trying to run a scam on him, and that there were twins and the one he saw before was my twin brother!" This man couldn't believe that his doctor would actually accuse him of running a scam. And there are other stories just like this one. These conventional doctors just don't want to believe that Dr. Berkson is curing people.

Another patient told me that the doctor he goes to in California told him that there was no way he could be getting any better. But this doctor thought it was Dr. Berkson who was "running a scam" on the patient, and just taking his money. But the patient told his doctor, "No, I'm really getting better." The doctor told him he couldn't be getting better, because "there is no cure for what you have." The patient told me he offered to show his doctor his blood test results, but the doctor didn't want to see them, because he was sure that Dr. Berkson's lab was "in on the scam!" But the patient said, "I'll go to your lab. Just tell me which lab to go to." So the doctor sent him to his own lab, and the patient went. And a few days later, the results came back, and of course, they were the same as the results Dr. Berkson's lab had gotten. I guess that doctor didn't care, because he still wasn't impressed.

Now, it's been almost eight years since I was first diagnosed with pancreatic cancer with metastases to the liver. And I'm feeling better than ever. So, I guess that, even though I wish other doctors would be more curious about Dr. Berkson and his non-toxic treatments, as long as patients keep finding out about him, and continue to be helped, that's what counts the most.

I find Paul's story very touching. I also find it very frightening, because I have no doubt, nor does he, that he'd be dead if he had listened to his more conventional doctors. I also chuckle when I read Paul's story. In addition to his wonderful tongue-in-cheek sense of humor, I admire his razor-sharp insights into conventional doctors' behavior and ways of thinking. What a shame it is that so many doctors who actually witness first-hand the success of treatments like the ones my contributors and I are writing about, dismiss what they actually see with their own eyes. Hopefully, more and more patients will "push the envelope," and help doctors to open their eyes to what they are actually witnessing, rather than dismissing these treatments as "anecdotal!"

I recently received an email from Paul. He wrote: "I am doing fine. I am an assistant scoutmaster of my son's Boy Scout troop. We went camping last weekend in nineteen-degree weather and light snow. We hiked part way up a mountain and had a blast." This from a man who began suffering the symptoms of pancreatic cancer eight years ago, and was told he'd be dead within four months!

The Ketogenic Diet

The Ketogenic Diet

Fasting and other dietary regimens have been used to treat epilepsy since biblical times. The ketogenic diet, which mimics the metabolism of fasting, was used by modern physicians to treat intractable epilepsy beginning in the 1920s. With the rising popularity of drug treatments, however, the ketogenic diet lost its previous status and was used in only a handful of clinics for most of the 20th century. The diet regained widespread recognition as a viable treatment option beginning in 1994 due to the efforts of parent advocate groups. Despite challenges to implementation of the treatment, the ketogenic diet has significant potential as a powerful tool for fighting epilepsy.
    —Elizabeth Thiele, MD, PhD
    Massachusetts General Hospital, 2006

Of the four treatments I am featuring in this book, the Ketogenic Diet has the distinction of having been around the longest. It is a very high fat, low carbohydrate diet that was first developed for the treatment of epilepsy at the Mayo Clinic in the 1920s, and went on to be championed at Johns Hopkins in Baltimore. Now many hospitals around the world are using it to treat children with epilepsy. But still, in the main, the medical community prefers to use anti-seizure drugs rather than the diet. In this section, you'll see why so many parents are upset about this—and why they think the diet should be the first line of defense against their children's seizures.

In addition to being the oldest of the four treatments featured in this book, the Ketogenic Diet is also the only one that has held a respected place in conventional medicine. In fact, before the advent of the newer anti-convulsant medications, the diet was one of the very few treatments known to work on seizures. There were a few medications, too: potassium bromide, developed in the late nineteenth and early twentieth centuries, and Phenobarbital, which came on the market in 1912. (http://en.wikipedia.org/wiki/Potassium_bromide; http://en.wikipedia.org/wiki/Phenobarbital)

In 1938, Dilantin was discovered, and after that, there was a huge emphasis on discovering other anti-convulsants that would be equally effective. In the 1940s, the use of the diet declined and became obsolete in most hospitals, but not at Hopkins. At Johns Hopkins, Dr. Samuel Livingston was a strong defender of the diet and continued to treat twenty to twenty-five patients a year, from 1937 until his retirement in the mid-1970s. But after Dr. Livingston retired, the numbers declined considerably.

In 1994, everything changed. Jim Abrahams, a Hollywood film writer/director/producer ("Airplane" and "Hot Shots"), became frustrated by the fact that his infant son, Charlie, who had a severe form of epilepsy, was continuing to deteriorate, despite numerous combinations of drugs and even one brain surgery. Finally, Jim did his own research and found that the Ketogenic Diet had been effective in stopping seizures in children like Charlie for over seventy years. Against his doctors' advice, Jim brought the then-20-month-old Charlie to Hopkins, and he was put on the diet.

Within forty-eight hours, Charlie's seizures were gone.

Both delighted and angry, Jim vowed to spend a major portion of the rest of his life spreading the word about the diet. He wanted to save other parents from the same unnecessary heartache he and his family had endured. For this purpose, he created The Charlie Foundation to Help Cure Pediatric Epilepsy: http://www.charliefoundation.org. Thanks to Jim and The Charlie Foundation, tens of thousands of children are now seizure-free.

Although the diet is now being administered in many hospitals around the world, I think it would have died out—to be totally replaced by anti-seizure medications—had Jim and Charlie not come along. I learned most of what I know about the diet from Jim. He also introduced me to the other parents whose stories I have included, and to the dietitians, as well.

As Dr. Elizabeth Thiele pointed out in the opening quote of this introduction, the idea that there is a relationship between food and seizures has been around for a very long time. In fact, the Hippocratic Corpus (c. 400 BC) proposed that dietary therapy was a sound treatment for epilepsy. (http://en.wikipedia.org/wiki/Ketogenic_diet#cite_note-Hippocrates2-12) The connection between fasting and stopping seizures was also recognized in the New Testament. The Book of Matthew mentions the connection: http://www.makingdisciplesforjesus.net/A%20Journey%20Through%20Matthew2/lesson17.htm. So does Mark 9:29: "This can come forth by nothing but by prayer and fasting." And the sixteenth century Italian painter Raphael depicted the child with seizures whom Jesus healed in his painting, "The Transfiguration" (1517): http://arthistoryfacts.com/Page8MyArtHistorySite.htm.

In the 1920s, the *Mayo Clinic Bulletin* gave an account of "favorable results of prolonged fasting reported from the Presbyterian Hospital in New York …" (http://honestmedicine.typepad.com/MayoBulletin_1921.pdf) Obviously, a person cannot fast forever and still live. So they proposed a very high fat, low carbohydrate diet that could mimic fasting in the body because it forces the body to burn fat, rather than sugar, for energy. In the 1920s, Dr. Russell Wilder of the Mayo Clinic named it the "Ketogenic Diet" because this kind of diet produces a substance called ketones, and a state called ketosis. In Chapter 8, ketogenic dietitian Milly Kelly describes the process very clearly. (Editor's note: For a more detailed description of the scientific basis for the diet, go to http://en.wikipedia.org/wiki/Ketogenic_diet. And for a more scholarly article, see "Clinical Aspects of the Ketogenic Diet," at http://site. matthewsfriends.org/uploads/pdf/HartmanViningKDReview.pdf.)

In this section, you'll hear from three parents, including Jim Abrahams (Chapter 7). In Chapter 9, Emma Williams, Matthew's mother, tells about how she begged her doctors in the UK to let her try the diet when Matthew was 2 years old, only to be turned down—even mocked. By the time she got their "permission" to try it, six years later, Matthew was already severely brain injured and physically disabled, as a result of years of seizures, as well as side effects from the medications he'd been taking. In 2004, Emma founded Matthew's Friends, the UK sister organization of The Charlie Foundation, to educate parents who want to try the diet, so that they won't have to go through what she and so many other parents have gone through. (http://site.matthewsfriends.org/)

In Chapter 10, you'll read the equally moving story of Jean McCawley's fight to get the Ketogenic Diet for her then-infant daughter, Julie. She succeeded after a year of trying. Unfortunately, by that time, Julie had been literally poisoned to near-death by the anti-seizure medication, Phenobarbital. The diet would have been a far better choice.

Neither parent was offered the diet; both had to fight for it.

With the diet, both Matthew and Julie improved immeasurably and almost instantaneously. Unfortunately, both children, now in their teens, have permanent disabilities resulting from both their pre-diet seizures and their pre-diet medications.

In Chapter 8, I depart from my usual format of one story per chapter, and have the two dietitians who championed the diet from 1948 to the present tell their stories. Millicent (Milly) Kelly was at Hopkins from 1948 to 1998. And Beth Zupec-Kania has worked with the diet from 1993 to the present. She developed the Keto-genic Diet program at Children's Hospital of Wisconsin (CHW) in

1993, and began working with The Charlie Foundation in 2006. She currently serves in two capacities: as Director of Programs for The Charlie Foundation, and as a part-time employee at CHW, providing backup to the primary ketogenic dietitian.

Ketogenic Diet Cost

The Ketogenic Diet costs much, much less than the majority of anti-seizure medications. As you can see by going to page 14 of the report, "Consumer Reports Best Buy Drugs: Treating Bipolar Disorder, Nerve Pain, and Fibromyalgia: The Anticonvulsants," the average oral anti-convulsant medication costs anywhere from $14 to $440 a month: http://www.consumerreports.org/health/resources/pdf/best-buy-drugs/Anticonvulsants-FINAL.pdf. (Editor's note: Prepared by *Consumer Reports*, this report lists anticonvulsants prescribed for fibromyalgia. I decided to include it here, nonetheless, because it contains the best comparative analysis I could find of the costs of such a wide array of anti-seizure drugs.) At the other end of the spectrum, and not included in this report, is ACTH, an injectable steroid used—until very recently—to control infantile spasms, at a cost of approximately $240,000 a month. Many of these anti-seizure medications have to be taken for the rest of the child's life.

The Ketogenic Diet is different in that children usually only need to be on it for approximately two years. After that, most can eat a regular diet and still maintain seizure control, with less or no medication. And Jim estimates that Charlie's food while on the diet cost no more or less than that of the other members of his family.

Because hospitalization is required at first to start a child on the diet, the cost of administering the diet is greatest in the very beginning. It is important that the diet be started under medical supervision. Foods must be prepared appropriately and measured carefully to ensure the correct proportion of fat, carbohydrate and protein.

The dietitian gives the parents the prescribed diet, and it is adjusted at various times throughout the child's life—for instance, during times of growth, as well as during times of illness. So parents will need the support of the dietitian at these times, as well. The diet works best when it is strictly adhered to.

The Ketogenic Diet has been found to improve 67 percent of the thousands of children with epilepsy who have had access to it since the 1920s. When appropriately supervised, its adverse effects are minimal, and the positive effects, in addition to improved seizure control and even a cure for epilepsy, include increased cognitive abilities, and improved disposition and development. Seventy percent of children have seizures controlled with medicine, but many of those come with debilitating side effects. Brain surgery, when appropriate, has tremendous cost, significant risk, and no guarantee of success. As you will see in the chapters that follow, early intervention with the Ketogenic Diet is essential, because seizures and medicine can cause irreparable damage.

Now, to Jim's story.

CHAPTER 7

Jim Abrahams

Charlie's Dad, Director of The Charlie Foundation to Help Cure Pediatric Epilepsy

IMPRESSION: It is my impression that Charlie has a mixed seizure disorder, most likely a variation of Lennox-Gastaut syndrome. Parents are fully aware of the ramifications of this diagnosis. Although there are many traditional combinations and permutations of drugs that could be used here, I agree with the current approach. It is my understanding that the next drug to be tried is a combination of Felbamate and Tegretol with which I have no problem. I would also consider the combination of Felbamate with Valproate with perhaps a benzodiazepine. In addition one wonders if the Felbamate could be pushed to an even higher dose than it is now, since we really do not know what the maximum dose of Felbamate is in young children. Another possibility is high dose Valproate monotherapy. One other alternative therapy which I have mentioned to the family, but only reluctantly because of the high incidence of side effects is high dose ACTH. The problem is that while high dose ACTH may be effective in stopping the seizures, they almost always recur as the dose is tapered. This makes one wonder if the risk-benefit ratio justifies the use of this somewhat dangerous mode of therapy. Finally, I think that if all pharmacological or therapeutic modalities fail, I would seriously consider a corpus colosotomy [an irreversible operation that severs the two halves of the brain] on this child. A corpus colosotomy would not be curative of all the seizure types, but may help the most troublesome part of his seizure complex, i.e. the drops.

— Written by Charlie's fourth pediatric neurologist, October 1993

Though it makes no mention of dietary therapy, two months after receiving this report, Charlie was seizure- and drug-free, thanks to the Ketogenic Diet.

For those of us who have had children with difficult-to-control epilepsy, it is quite literally impossible to put the feelings into words. Sadness, frustration, agony, helplessness, anger, pain, despair. These words, even when bunched together, fall short. It's not just the seizures, or the drug side effects, or the failed surgeries. It's standing by and watching your child slip away—watching the lights go out—one day, one hour, one minute at a time.

That's how it was with my son, Charlie. His first seizure was on his first birthday, March 11, 1993. Over the following months he tried every available anticonvulsant drug medication. The seizures got worse. Dozens, frequently as many as a hundred per day. Brain surgery didn't work either.

For me, the hardest part of Charlie's seizures was seeing his eyes. One minute they were bright, clear, smiley. A split second later they were dull, unfocused … dead. Then they'd roll back. It was like watching him die. The rest of the seizure, whether it was a quick drop or his body stiffening and shaking with a high piercing noise, was terrifying and heartbreaking. But, for some reason, what has stuck with me the most were his eyes. No matter how many times we saw them, it never got easier for Nancy and me.

We were deep into the drug regimens when our neurologist told us the best chance to stop the seizures would be a surgery to drain fluid from Charlie's left ventricle. Turns out that seizures don't emanate from the ventricles of the brain, but we trusted him and his credentials. Charlie weighed about eighteen pounds on the day of the surgery. They promised Nancy he'd be asleep when they took him into surgery. But he was wide awake and crying when she had to hand him over. We were told the "procedure" was relatively simple, painless, and would last less than an hour. Three excruciating hours later, someone came up to the waiting room and told us that Charlie was having a bad reaction to the morphine, and that we needed to wait a little longer.

"Morphine?!" we asked. "For what?"

"Pain."

"How much pain?"

"It's hard to tell. He was uncomfortable."

"What was the bad reaction?"

"Hives."

When we finally were allowed to see him in the recovery room he was all red and puffy. Two days later, after we left the hospital, his seizures returned.

Charlie saw four pediatric neurologists in three cities. Over nine months, the seizures that had begun so subtly mounted in severity and frequency into the thousands. The seemingly endless drugs and drug cocktails altered his personality, development, appetite, sleep, complexion and bowels. We watched helplessly as he began to fade away. The fourth neurologist, quoted above, basically told us his epilepsy was incurable—that Charlie could expect a life of seizures and "progressive retardation." Nancy and I had to pull the car over on the way home from his announcement of hopelessness because we could not see through our tears.

Then, in an effort to figure out how Charlie and his brother and sister and Nancy and I were going to get through the rest of his life with such a bleak prognosis, I went to the UCLA medical library (those were pre-Internet days) to do some reading. Again, this was not in an effort to find a cure—after all, we had taken Charlie to many of the leading experts in the country, and they had all concurred: Medications and surgery were the only alternatives.

I went to the library to figure out how our family was going to cope with what we were told lay ahead of us.

Neither science nor research come naturally to me, but here is a sampling of the medical information I found—reports and studies about the Ketogenic Diet—on that one day in the medical library at UCLA in the fall of 1993. What confused me the most was that for years—even generations—the Ketogenic Diet had been consistently reported as helping a majority of the thousands of children who had tried it. Yet, though they all knew about the diet, not one of Charlie's doctors had even mentioned it to us.

> "Thirty-seven patients with essential epilepsy have been treated for periods of from three to thirty months by means of a ketogenic diet. Twelve have improved and nineteen have been free from attacks since institution of this treatment. Three patients remained free from convulsions for three to eight months and were not heard from again."
>
> *New England Journal of Medicine*, M. G. Peterman, MD, Mayo Clinic, April 4, 1925.

~

> "Of thirty patients treated with the ketogenic diet, 26.6 percent have remained free from attacks for long periods and have resumed an unrestricted diet."
>
> "Epilepsy in Childhood—Results With the Ketogenic Diet," Lawson Wilkins, MD, *The Journal of Pediatrics*, January through June, 1937.

~

> "Results of treatment with ketogenic diet in 530 cooperative patients: No known attacks 5 to 36 years: 162 (30.6%); Improvement: 128 (24.1%); Failure 206 [38.9%]."
>
> *Convulsive Disorders in Children—With Reference to Treatment with Ketogenic Diet*, Dr. Haddow M. Keith, Mayo Clinic, 1963.

~

> "As of 1958, we had treated 426 children with the ketogenic diet. Seizures were controlled in 52%; in an additional 27%

there was marked improvement; 21% did not respond to treatment. Since 1958 we have treated an additional 575 patients with the ketogenic diet regimen and the results relative to seizure control were essentially the same as those reported previously."

> *Comprehensive Management of Epilepsy in Infancy, Childhood and Adolescence.* Samuel Livingston, Johns Hopkins, 1972.

"Before using the ketogenic diet, 80% of the patients had multiple seizure types and 88% were treated with multiple antiepileptic drugs; these children were among our most intractable patients. Thirty-eight percent of these children had a decrease in seizure frequency of at least 50% and 29% had virtually complete seizure control."

> *Efficacy of the Ketogenic Diet for Intractable Seizure Disorders: Review of 58 Cases*, Kinsman, Vining, Quaskey, Mellitis, Freeman, Johns Hopkins, 1992.

Astonishingly, the above-quoted 1992 article had been published in *Epilepsia,* the premiere medical epilepsy journal, just a year before Charlie got sick. It was hot off the presses. It was the state of the art. It was presented at the Child Neurology and American Epilepsy Society meetings in 1992. Okay, one of the neurologists who saw Charlie might have missed it. Maybe even two. But all four? How could that possibly be? Did they all miss it, and the seven decades of evidence that preceded it, or did they dismiss it? Eighteen years later, I'm still asking these questions. Back in 1993, when, as a result of my research, I broached the subject to Charlie's primary neurologist and mentioned the Ketogenic Diet and another possibility we were considering—an herbalist we had heard about who worked out of a strip mall in Houston, Texas—he said, "Flip a coin, I don't believe either will work." For the final time, we took his advice. We flipped the coin. It said to go to Texas. We did, and Charlie's seizures continued.

At last I called Dr. John Freeman from Johns Hopkins, one of the authors of the 1992 article, and co-author of the book, *Seizures and Epilepsy in Childhood: A Parent's Guide.* He suggested we bring Charlie to Hopkins. We did and Charlie was started on the diet. He went from having dozens, frequently as many as one hundred seizures a day, to zero within forty-eight hours. He was off his four anti-convulsant medicines within a month. Five years later he was weaned off the diet and has remained seizure- and drug-free while eating a regular diet to this day.

What makes Charlie's story unusual is not that his seizures were difficult to control, or that medications had bad side effects and failed to help. The truth is that about thirty percent of children with epilepsy do not have their seizures controlled by drugs. According to the organization, Citizens United for Research in Epilepsy (CURE), "It is estimated that close to 2 of the 3 million Americans with epilepsy do not have complete seizure control, or only experience seizure control at the cost of debilitating side effects from medications."

Think about it. As I quoted earlier, Dr. Peterman from the Mayo Clinic first reported the Ketogenic Diet's extraordinary success in 1925. In the following decades there were dozens of reports from a variety of hospitals with stunningly similar results. How many children, worldwide, have suffered unnecessarily because their parents were uninformed or misinformed about the diet since 1925? What is the collateral damage? It's a human tragedy of incalculable proportions.

What *does* make Charlie's story unusual was that he eventually got to the Ketogenic Diet. Though it had been a first-line therapy for children with intractable epilepsy in the 1930s and '40s in America, it began to fall into disuse when anti-convulsant medications came along. By the time we took Charlie to Hopkins in 1993, the diet was on the verge of extinction. Hopkins had one of two or three Ketogenic Diet programs in the world, and they were only initiating a handful of children every year.

Later, when we asked Charlie's neurologists why they hadn't told us about the diet, these were the answers:

1. "The Ketogenic Diet is a high-fat diet and therefore may have health consequences."
2. "The Ketogenic Diet is too difficult."
3. "I've never seen it work."
4. "There is no science behind the diet."

Because I feel each of these arguments exposes an important element of a system badly derailed, I'd like to address them individually.

1. Health consequences? As the quote that begins this chapter indicates, Charlie's doctors were considering several extremely dangerous treatment options: yet more drugs and drug combinations in higher doses, with terrible side effects; ACTH, a brutal, multi-thousand dollar per day injected hormone therapy; and cutting his brain in half, i.e. a corpus colosotomy. This surgery is irreversible and precludes any possibility of a normal life—or even seizure freedom. The safest, most effective option for Charlie—the Ketogenic Diet—wasn't even discussed.

2. Too difficult? Shouldn't that be the family's decision? Is the standard of care really that a practitioner can decide what therapy is "too difficult" for a critically sick child's parents to undertake? Nancy and I assumed a system of informed joint decision making between physician and patient. We were wrong.

3. I've never seen it work? What is the point of constant medical meetings and relentless publications if each physician needs to see evidence firsthand? Especially when, as I have demonstrated, there existed a strong predisposition to ignore dietary therapy. How's that for a Catch-22? "I'm not going to believe the Ketogenic Diet works until I see it in my practice, but I'm not going to try it."

4. No science? I find this the most insidious of all the arguments. There is zero science behind any of the drugs or drug combinations Charlie had been prescribed. Zero. It is illegal to scientifically study medications in children younger than four. Plus there is no science behind the effects of endless drug combinations on people of any age. To arbitrarily represent that medications are science, and to use that misrepresentation as an argument against the Ketogenic Diet, is a cruel double standard. In fact, statistically, after the failure of two medications, the diet has a far greater chance of success than any medication or combination of medications.

I found myself in an extraordinary position. I had experienced the horror of Charlie's childhood epilepsy. I had stumbled across a dying medical therapy that could benefit most and cure many—but that somehow, unfathomably, did not fit the model and constraints of modern Western medicine. And I knew that Charlie was but one of millions of children who were in the same position. So, Nancy and I started The Charlie Foundation to Help Cure Pediatric Epilepsy in order to elevate awareness: www.charliefoundation.org.

At its inception in 1994, The Charlie Foundation certainly had a clear idea of what we wanted to accomplish, but there was no road map. So we adopted a sort of "if you build it, they will come" attitude. We decided to try a two-pronged approach, focusing on both public and medical awareness.

Knowing the incredible power of parent- and patient-driven movements, as well as the desperation of parents who walked in our shoes, we first dedicated ourselves to a campaign of public awareness. My background in the movie industry proved valuable here. We produced a forty-five-minute video hosted by our friend Meryl Streep, entitled "An Introduction to the Ketogenic Diet." (To date we've distributed over 250,000 copies.) As a result, Charlie's story was picked up by the media. Charlie and the Ketogenic Diet were featured in *People Magazine,* "Dateline NBC" (on three occasions), "Entertainment Tonight," *USA Today, The Wall Street Journal, Newsweek* and countless other periodicals. We were reaching the public.

Because the diet had been in existence for so many years, we began to hear from other families who had had success with the Ketogenic Diet. One of the stories that was particularly dramatic occurred in 1975. Connie Intermitte wrote us about how her then-4-year-old son Tim had gained seizure- and drug-freedom with the diet—but not until her family was forced to go through incredible measures. With her permission and input, in 1998 we made an ABC television movie, "First Do No Harm," starring Meryl Streep. Millions watched.

At the same time we worked through the scientific and medical communities in an effort to facilitate research into the diet's mechanisms and knowledge of its application. To that end, we sponsored meetings among physicians and dietitians and helped support research.

We have held, and continue to hold, educational events for professionals. From our first seminar in September 1995, which was attended by over one hundred neurologists, dietitians and nurses, to our first-ever International Symposium on Dietary Therapies for Epilepsy and Other Neurological Disorders in 2008, and our Dietitians and Nurses Forum in 2009, our efforts have never slowed.

Awareness ticked dramatically upward. Other parents and parent groups began to spring up around the world. Other families came forth with their success stories. In 2007, Dr. Deborah Snyder, whose son, Bryce, became seizure- and drug-free on the Ketogenic Diet, wrote her book, *Keto Kid.* In it she outlines her positive attitude toward the diet, describing the empowering aspects as her family participated in Bryce's cure. At the same time she debunks the medical establishment's boilerplate "too difficult" argument against the diet.

In 2006, Beth Zupec-Kania, RD, CD, who had been working with the Ketogenic Diet since 1993, joined The Charlie Foundation, and has thus far visited over seventy hospitals around the world teaching the team approach to dietary therapy.

Matthew's Friends, a sister organization in England, began in 2004 when Emma Williams' son Matthew was finally offered the diet, six years after she saw "First Do No Harm," and began asking for it. He attained over 90 percent seizure reduction. But by then Matthew had experienced substantial irreversible brain damage from the years of pummeling by seizures and drugs. Among many other activities, Matthew's Friends hosted the Second Global Symposium on Dietary Therapy for Epilepsy and Other Neurological Disorders in Scotland in October 2010. This charity has had a significant impact on the world of dietary therapy for epilepsy.

In Japan in 2007, Hiroyuki Nakatsuta started a similar group based on his son's success with the diet. Veronica and Helmut Blum initiated Ciros Centrum in Austria in 2008 after their son, Ciro, became drug- and seizure-free on the Ketogenic Diet. Earlier this year, 2010, Avery Osgood's parents, Jennifer and John, started Avery's Alliance in Denver, Colorado after his seizures disappeared, thanks to the diet. And in March 2010, Paulette George published her book, *Good Morning Beautiful*, about how the diet helped her daughter, Christina, gain seizure freedom.

Blogs, chat rooms, and other support groups have sprung up worldwide.

The diet itself has been refined in terms of initiation, reduced adverse effects and palatability. As doctors and dietitians implemented the diet over the years, they developed pre-diet screening procedures to ensure safety and rule out metabolic contraindications, as well as side effects that would interfere with efficacy. Hospitals have developed a team approach in which neurologists, dietitians, nurses and pharmacologists collaborate on the diet as it is applied to each new patient. Dietary supplements have been added prophylactically to ensure nutritional adequacy and to prevent constipation, the most common adverse effect of the diet. Two new versions of the diet were developed—the Low Glycemic Index Treatment and the Modified Atkins Diet—less restrictive diets for older children and adults. New infant formulas have made the diet accessible to infants and tube-fed children.

As the diet has grown in awareness, popularity and understanding, it is beginning to be used with other neurological disorders. Some patients with ALS, early onset Alzheimer's disease, Parkinson's disease, and even malignant brain tumors have improved dramatically with the Ketogenic Diet.

Our progress was summarized in a June 17, 2009 article published in *The Journal of Child Neurology:*

> The past 15 years have witnessed an enormous growth of interest in the ketogenic diet. At this writing, a PubMed search indicates that nearly 750 peer-reviewed articles on the ketogenic diet have been published since 1994. In 2006, symposia at both the International Child Neurology Association and Child Neurology Society annual meetings were the first sessions ever held devoted solely to the ketogenic diet. In April

2008, a 4-day international conference devoted to the use of dietary treatments brought 270 attendees to Phoenix, Arizona. The ketogenic diet is now available in over 50 countries, in all continents except Antarctica. As a direct result of this growing interest, an expert consensus guideline was commissioned by The Charlie Foundation, written by 26 neurologists and dietitians from 9 countries, endorsed by the Child Neurology Society, and published in *Epilepsia* in November, 2008. This consensus guideline was designed not only to suggest the optimal management of children receiving the ketogenic diet but also to highlight aspects of dietary treatments that were unclear and potentially areas of future research.

—Dr. Eric Kossoff, Beth Zupec-Kania, RD, Dr. Jong Rho

One year earlier, in 2008, Dr. Helen Cross from Great Ormond Hospital in London published a Class 1 randomized double-blind study concluding: "Forty-two percent of children with epilepsy who were following a Ketogenic Diet for three months had a greater than 50 percent reduction in seizure frequency with 19 percent reporting a reduction in seizures of 75 percent or more."

With this study, Dr. Cross has taken a significant step toward gaining medical acceptance of the Ketogenic Diet, while, at the same time, successfully removing the credibility of the "no science" argument.

Today, there are over 150 hospitals worldwide with Ketogenic Diet programs. The Charlie Foundation to Help Cure Pediatric Epilepsy has sponsored and run over 125 Ketogenic Diet seminars and training programs, and has been involved in the publication of six books. Our website, www.charliefoundation.org, is a comprehensive source of Ketogenic Diet resources, including medical opinions, a list of Ketogenic Diet FAQs, keto centers, diet implementation, recipes, other families' stories and chat rooms. We will be hosting the Global Symposium for Dietary Therapies in 2012 and are in the planning stages with a local university hospital for a Charlie Foundation Dietary Therapy Center, which promises to be the gold standard of Ketogenic Diet implementation in the Western United States.

Most importantly, thousands of children have gotten better.

So, I don't want this chapter to read like I'm some angry parent who's still grinding his axe eighteen years later. Every day we are overwhelmingly grateful for getting Charlie back, and every day we are overjoyed to hear from other parents who have now had the same experience, in part because of Charlie.

But sadly, as I write this chapter, there remains a vast majority of children who could benefit from the Ketogenic Diet whose parents never hear about it, are talked out of it, or have it implemented too late, or improperly. We hear from them daily. The disconnect between good health and other influences in Western medicine is blatant. In surveys among pediatric neurologists, only a small percent use dietary therapy. The primary explanation they give today is the absence of access to dietitians who are trained in administering the Ketogenic Diet. Yet, for reasons incomprehensible to me, they rarely refer patients to the many well known Ketogenic Diet centers that do exist.

A few days ago, I visited Steele Schaaf, a beautiful 7-year-old Southern California boy who had started the Ketogenic Diet six weeks earlier. Steele had been suffering severe daily epilepsy for four years; eight medications and a vagal nerve stimulator implant had failed to help. For years his parents were not told about the Ketogenic Diet. Finally a doctor mentioned it to them during one of Steele's many trips to the emergency room. As of today Steele has had one seizure in the past ten days. That happened when he "cheated" on his diet and had a cookie. His parents are overjoyed at his increased cognitive improvement and disposition, not to mention the absence of seizures. His mom told me, "We've got him back."

In 2008, medical guidelines were published advocating that the "KD should be strongly considered after the failure of two or three medications regardless of age or gender." This was considered a giant step forward for a therapy that had been largely considered a "last resort."

But it's not enough:

1. Statistically, after the failure of a single anti-epileptic medication there is a 10-15 percent chance a second medication will stop seizures and only a 20 percent chance drugs will ever work. As we've already seen, the Ketogenic Diet has a much higher success rate. Why wouldn't you "strongly consider" the therapy that is safest and has the greatest chance of success?

2. Early intervention is essential. Seizures and drugs damage young brains. Trying a new medication means slowly titrating the dosage to a therapeutic level, waiting to see if it's effective (or if it becomes toxic); then, if it is ineffective or becomes toxic, slowly weaning off. The process can take months. Two or three medications, and the accompanying seizures that take place when the medications don't work, may already have done irreparable damage. There is no telling at what point during these assaults on Charlie's one-year-old brain that his autism was triggered. There's no telling at what point Matthew Williams started suffering irreversible injuries. We know for a fact that Julie McCawley was blinded by a drug reaction to the first antiepileptic medication she took.

There can be no dispute that if these three children, and hundreds of thousands like them, had been offered the Ketogenic Diet as a first line therapy, their lives would not have been needlessly damaged.

What is the point of real evidence-based medicine when the evidence is ignored? What happened to "… first do no harm?"

I have great admiration for anyone who would choose to spend his or her life helping children with neurological disorders. Pediatric neurology is very low on the "glitz scale"; it's toward the bottom of the medical specialties list in terms of financial rewards; the responsibility and dedication must feel overwhelming. The neurologists and epileptologists on The Charlie Foundation's scientific advisory board, as well as so many others I've met over the years, are among the most dedicated people I know.

So I do not feel that what happened to Charlie and countless other children like him is due to any one, or a handful, of practitioners. I strongly believe that in this pocket of Western medicine where I have spent the last eighteen years and about which I feel qualified to comment, there has been a pervasive systemic failure. As we all learned during the recent health care debate (2010), medicine rewards tests, procedures and medications rather than real success with patients. Dietary therapy, though successful, is time intensive and not remunerative.

Hospitals are businesses. They have to earn profits. EEGs, other tests and surgeries are not just the bread and butter of most neurology departments; they are the meat and potatoes.

Additionally, when we look at the underuse of the diet, we cannot overestimate the role that is played by physicians' susceptibility to the influence of the pharmaceutical companies. Certainly Charlie's primary neurologist was incredibly candid when he was asked on "Dateline NBC" about Charlie and the Ketogenic Diet:

Dateline NBC: "Why are modern doctors ignoring this diet? Charlie's own doctor has a surprising answer."

Charlie's Neurologist: "There's no big drug company behind the Ketogenic Diet and there probably never can be unless somebody starts marketing sausage and eggs with cream sauce on it as a drug."

Dateline NBC: "You're saying that, in a sense, one of the reasons that the Ketogenic Diet is not popular at this point is that there's not a big drug company behind it selling it to the doctors?"

Charlie's Neurologist: "I think that's probably true. I hate to say that. But I think that's probably true."

The entire interview can be seen on our website at www. charliefoundation.org.

This is an urgent and enormous problem. According to Citizens United for Research in Epilepsy (CURE), "Epilepsy affects over three million Americans of all ages—more than multiple sclerosis, cerebral palsy, muscular dystrophy and Parkinson's disease combined. Almost 500 new cases of epilepsy are diagnosed every day in the U.S. and epilepsy affects 50,000,000 people worldwide." To understand that there is a perfected, readily available dietary therapy that can and does help a majority of the children who have had access to it, yet is unknown or unavailable to most, is a brutal commentary on today's modern Western healthcare system.

So, beyond promoting public and medical awareness of a therapy that fits like a square peg in the round hole of Western medicine, The Charlie Foundation has added a new message. We feel it is necessary for each of us to become active participants in our children's medical destinies. Today, among our top priorities, is empowering parents with the information they need to trust their instincts and battle for their children. There is a tendency when we walk into a doctor's office to want to hand over our problem and say, "Here it is; please fix it." It's comfortable, it's easy, and more often than not, it works. Just as we take comfort in deferring to them, many doctors are unwilling to confide in us that we may have stepped into one of Western medicine's black holes. Clearly, most children with difficult-to-control seizures have stepped into one of them.

What does this mean? It means that our medical problems and our children's medical problems are precisely that—ours. At first, that's a pretty intimidating and perhaps a seemingly foolish concept, both to us and to some physicians. After all, they went through years of education. They've seen countless patients in their practices. And then we walk into their offices with a disease we probably don't even know how to spell. How presumptuous and perhaps foolish of us, the parents, to ask and then pursue the hard questions, learn the side effects, get the second opinions, do the research, and participate in the cure—in short, to become proactive. Ironically, the "side effect" of participating in our own medical destinies and those of our children may not only lead to getting better sooner. It is also empowering. Though I would do almost anything to go back and have Charlie not suffer epilepsy, the experience has been empowering. Regardless of whether responsibility for informing ourselves confirms what we learn from our physicians, it's nevertheless empowering to become informed.

We take control of so many lesser issues in our families' lives—meals, bedtimes, TV hours—why not have that same attitude with the most important issue, our families' health? In the worst case, we have learned something new; in the best case, we have improved both our lives and the lives of our children. Isn't that each of our ultimate missions?

I am frankly in awe of Jim for his years-long, day-in-and-day-out dedication to helping parents who want the diet for their children to get it. Jim has read letters to me from parents who were told—wrongly—by their doctors that the diet would not work for their children, and that even if it might work, it would be just too difficult to administer. Jim helps each and every parent he can help—even though it brings back such painful memories for him—and even visits many of these children. And in several instances, especially in cases where the diet is being administered incorrectly, he calls hospital personnel to help them get on the right track. Without Jim, I am positive the diet would have died.

As you will see from Chapters 9 and 10, both Emma Williams and Jean McCawley are sure they never would have learned about the diet without Jim. This is true of thousands of other parents, as well.

But first, in Chapter 8, you will hear from two of the dietitians who have championed the diet since 1948.

Two "Keto Dietitians"

The Ketogenic Diet wouldn't be here today if it were not for the tireless work of several doctors, nurses, dietitians and parents. Most of the chapters about the Ketogenic Diet in this book are written by parents. Here, in this chapter, I am including the words of the two dietitians who have also labored very hard to keep the diet alive.

Their words also provide us with lots of history about this diet. For more historical information about the diet, please consult the Appendix.

Millicent Kelly, RD:
Dietitian at Johns Hopkins
from 1948-1998

That Milly Kelly was at Johns Hopkins from 1948 to 1998 is amazing in itself. But equally amazing is the fact that she worked under the two doctors who were the diet's most ardent medical champions there: Samuel Livingston, MD and John Freeman, MD.

Milly is a legend. For this reason, I was more than a bit intimidated at the prospect of approaching her. Although I had to track her down (she was in the process of relocating from Maryland to North Carolina), Milly couldn't have been more wonderful: so easy to talk to and so enthusiastic about participating in any book that would make the Ketogenic Diet available to more children. Like most of the other people who have contributed chapters, I now consider Milly to be a very good friend.

Milly's section contains the best description of the diet itself, and how it works, that I have ever read. I think you will agree that in this chapter, Milly reveals her wonderful combination of sweetness, love and determination.

It is my honor to introduce her now.

In her words …

Following my graduation from the University of North Carolina at Greensboro in 1948, I was fortunate to be accepted into the fall dietary internship at the Johns Hopkins Hospital School of Dietetics. Upon completing my internship, I automatically became a member of the American Dietetic Association. At that time, to be a member of the ADA, and to be able to practice as a full-fledged dietitian, you needed either an internship, or a master's degree, or three years working in an accredited hospital.

The Hopkins internship was a one-year program that went from September 1, 1948 through August 31, 1949. We were on duty six days a week from 6 a.m. to 6 p.m. On our one day off, we often attended classes, taught by the doctors and dietitians. From the dietitians we learned about the different diets we would be preparing for patients, including low salt diets, low sugar diets, diets for patients with diabetes, and of course, the Ketogenic Diet for children with epilepsy. This is where I first learned about the Ketogenic Diet. And the doctors taught us about the diseases specific to the diets we were learning to prepare.

When I came to Hopkins, the Ketogenic Diet was already in full use, under the direction of Dr. Samuel Livingston, Professor in Pediatrics and Director of the Epilepsy Clinic. Dr. Livingston really championed the diet, and came to be called the Father of the Ketogenic Diet. He worked at Hopkins for nearly forty years, from 1937 until his retirement in the mid-1970s.

Dr. Livingston was amazingly brilliant and devoted to the diet and to his patients. For example, he knew that many of his patients would find it difficult to return to Hopkins for their follow-up appointments. So he would travel throughout the country, setting up an office in his hotel room in different cities, where he would see his patients. That shows you how special he was.

When I completed my dietary internship, I was asked to remain on the staff at Hopkins. My first job was as a Nutrition Instructor to the JHH School of Nursing, a three-year degree program. Only college graduates were accepted into this program—quite a change from today's requirements for becoming a nurse, which are much less stringent. I taught there for about ten years, instructing the nursing students about the Ketogenic Diet, as well as the diets for every other condition requiring a special diet.

Later, I transferred to the Nutrition Department, and was assigned to the Nutrition Clinic, which was staffed by four dietitians. (Special credit should go to one of these dietitians, in particular: Gloria Elfert, my teacher, my mentor and friend, for her work with the Ketogenic Diet.) Our function was to teach the patients whose conditions required a special diet—both inpatients and outpatients—and to give them special dietary instruction so they would be able to prepare their meals correctly at home. We instructed them in just about every kind of diet: diabetic, weight loss, low sodium, low cholesterol, high fiber, etc.

The Ketogenic Diet was very popular at that time, and all four of us were proficient with it. Through the years, dietitians came and went, and when I finally retired for the first time in the fall of 1990, I was the only dietitian remaining who was skilled with it.

When the diet was first used in the 1930s and 1940s, only a few drugs were available. Also, back then, foods were pure, devoid of nitrates, and there were very few canned, packaged and processed foods with additives on the market. But then, as more drugs became available, many doctors either didn't believe in the diet, questioned its nutritional adequacy, or opted to prescribe drugs. And so, there was a decline in the use of the diet in most of the hospitals that had Ketogenic Diet programs. But not at Hopkins.

Dr. Livingston's results were phenomenal. He published a paper in 1972 describing the 1,001 patients he treated with the diet during his nearly forty years at JHH. Fifty-two percent experienced full seizure control, and 27 percent significantly improved. What drug company today can make such claims? (Editor's note: See details on these claims on Table 2, page 44 of the chapter, "History and Origin of the Ketogenic Diet," from *Epilepsy and the Ketogenic Diet*, edited by C. E. Stafstrom and J. M. Rho. http://tinyurl. com/27880bf)

Dr. Livingston had wonderful, devoted dietitians as helpers; I learned under the masters. Those dedicated dietitians compiled by hand the exchange lists that were used in calculating the diet, years before calculators, computers and "Bowes and Church" were ever thought of. (Editor's note: *Food Values of Portions Commonly Used*, by Anna De Planter Bowes and Helen Nichols Church, is a resource book in wide use now for calculating the makeup of just about every known food—broken down into weight [in grams], protein, fats, carbohydrates, and vitamins and minerals. http://www.amazon.com/ Bowes-Churchs-Values-Portions-Commonly/dp/0397554354) These exchange lists are still in use today, with some modifications.

Some people think that any diet, merely high in fat and low in carbohydrates, is automatically ketogenic. It isn't. The Ketogenic Diet must be calculated accurately to a tenth of a gram. Since each food on the diet has to be prepared according to carefully planned guidelines and weighed on a gram scale (in one-gram increments), these lists and books include amounts (in grams) of protein, fat and carbohydrates in a given weight (in grams) of various foods in various categories. We have books, calculators and computers now. But back then, this was all done by hand—a method I continued to use as long as I worked with patients on the diet.

The diet was individualized for each child for their particular nutritional needs. It is still this way today. So each child does not get the same diet. To figure out what their nutritional needs are, you weigh them and take their height, and you then compare that to the chart, which tells you what a healthy child at a certain percentile should weigh, and how tall he or she should be. Then you adjust their calories accordingly. If they're underweight, you'll want them to gain weight slowly. If they're overweight, you'll want them to lose weight.

For the diet to work—to stop or lessen seizures—children have to stay in what is known as ketosis, which means that their body starts burning fat for energy, instead of using carbohydrates. So we keep the carbohydrates very, very low.

The Ketogenic Diet has sound reasoning behind it. Normally, the body burns starches and sugars (glucose) as its main sources of energy, but it can only store a 24-48 hour supply. When glucose has been depleted, and is no longer available for energy production—as is the case with the Ketogenic Diet—the body begins to draw on its other energy components: fats and proteins. This forces the body and brain to switch from burning glucose to burning fat for energy. (The body uses protein for growth and repair.) When such a high fat, low carbohydrate diet is eaten, it results in the accumulation of waste materials (called ketone bodies) that build up in the blood and urine, mimicking the same substances that are metabolized from the body of a fasting person. These ketone bodies, which build up in the blood and spill over into the urine, produce an anticonvulsant effect, tending to inhibit seizures.

The value of fasting in seizure control has been known for centuries, although the exact mechanism of the diet is not understood.

Because the diet allows a patient to remain in a constant state of ketosis, just like one who is fasting, it became known as the Ketogenic Diet. Ketone bodies not only act as a sedative, they also have an appetite-suppressing effect. Ketosis allows the child to be more alert, with greater clarity of thought than when in a medicated state. It also gives rise to a distinctive fruity odor to the breath—called "ketone breath." This is an easy way to check for ketosis.

Starting a child on the Ketogenic Diet requires a great deal of advance planning and the cooperation of so many people: the child's family, pediatric neurologists and epileptologists, staff nurses, dietary and pharmacy staff. For the diet to be successful, it also requires a commitment for follow-up at home for a period of one to two years. (After two years, most children are able to eat a normal diet.)

Educating the patient and the family to prepare acceptable meals at home, and to adhere to the prescribed rules, is extremely time-consuming. Everyone involved needs to understand the purpose of the diet, the importance of following the diet exactly as prescribed, and the precision with which it is calculated. The child must receive sufficient calories for energy and maintenance of growth, and the calorie allowance must be distributed according to a prescribed ratio. The dietitian calculates meal plans to satisfy individual food preferences, according to the dietary prescription. Modifications in calories are made as needed to meet growth and activity requirements.

When I was at Hopkins, this preparation period was intense. Even before the child was hospitalized to begin the diet, the dietitian had already contacted the family, filled out an information sheet, getting lots of information: birth date, age, height, weight, eating habits, food likes and dislikes, food allergies, etc. Before the child arrived at Hopkins, we had calculated his or her individual diet and created at least twelve meal plans for him or her. On the day before admission, the patient and family attended class in the outpatient pediatric seizure clinic with a Ketogenic Diet consultant. The routine was explained. The family was given various handouts and the twelve meal plans for when the child went home.

During the time the child was hospitalized to begin the diet, the parents went through a very rigorous training program, where we taught them how to use the gram scale, and exactly how to prepare ketogenic meals for their children when they went home. (Editor's note: Please see the Appendix for more precise information on the details of this rigorous training program, as well as precise details about exactly how the diet is generally introduced to the child during his or her hospitalization.)

This kind of precise parent education and administration of the diet went on for the entire time I was at Hopkins, because when Dr. Livingston retired in 1976, he was replaced by another doctor who was dedicated to the diet: Dr. John Freeman from Stanford. Dr. Freeman had attended medical school at JHH, where he learned about the Ketogenic Diet. He believed in it, and it was my understanding that he came back to Hopkins because of the diet. So the dietitians in the Nutrition Clinic continued to hone their skills in the preparation and teaching of the Ketogenic Diet under Dr. Freeman's tutelage. We were admitting ten to fifteen new patients per year, more or less.

Gradually, the original dietitians left for other jobs or retired, and by 1996, I was the only dietitian remaining at Hopkins with enough knowledge and experience to do the diet.

When I retired for the first time on August 31, 1990, Dr. Freeman asked me to stay on until he could find a replacement. I agreed, and became a part-time Ketogenic Diet consultant in the hospital on those days when patients were in his care. I did this for two years, without salary, until a paid fee schedule was set up. This didn't bother me at all. I loved my work so much that it added a great deal to my life, even without pay!

Some people think that I started the diet. But I didn't. It started back in the 1920s and 1930s. I just worked with it and was faithful and loyal to my patients and their families. Through the years, I taught dietitians, student dietitians, nurses and student nurses the mechanics of the diet. I consider myself to be a very simple and humble person, with a heart full of love for God's children with epilepsy and for their parents. Dr. Freeman actually paid me a huge compliment in 1994, on "Dateline NBC," when he said, "Without Milly, the diet would be gone … it's that simple." He said the same thing at the first International Conference in Phoenix in 2008.

Then, in 1993, everything changed when Jim Abrahams, a movie producer, brought his 20-month-old son Charlie to Hopkins to start the Ketogenic Diet. Charlie had endured seizures for almost a year, and Jim and his wife Nancy had spent a fortune going from one doctor to another. Nothing helped, and Charlie's seizures worsened, despite an incredible array of drugs and drug combinations, thousands of blood draws, MRIs, EEGs, CAT scans, PET scans, a brain surgery, four pediatric neurologists in three states, two homeopathic doctors, one faith healer, countless prayers and indescribable agony. By the time he came to us, Charlie could not walk, talk or sit up. In just forty-eight hours after starting the diet—BINGO!—his seizures stopped entirely.

Jim was amazed—and angry. He could not understand why the diet was not better known, and he couldn't do enough to make sure other families would not have to endure the unnecessary suffering and agony that he and his family had gone through. A man of vision, Jim was determined to tell the whole world about this miracle so that children with seizures could be helped. And ever since then, this humble, modest, talented, unselfish and generous man has devoted his life to raising money for awareness of epilepsy, and of this simple dietary cure for it. He is an amazing man. He cares deeply for his family, he loves children, and is concerned for all mankind. He is human to the bone.

Then, because of Jim, in 1994, "Dateline NBC," one of the most popular television programs, featured Charlie's story. After that, things just exploded. All the phones at Hopkins were jammed, with people calling from all over the United States requesting appointments—over 500 the first day—and they continued all week long, and for years thereafter. The storm had begun.

Our staff was small, consisting of Dr. Freeman and his associate, Dr. Ilene Vining, who replaced Dr. Freeman when he retired, and is there to this day as head of the clinic; Dr. Freeman's coordinator/counselor, Diana Pillas, who made the appointments and was so nurturing to families; the nurse, Jane Casey, a secretary and me. That was it. We all went to work double overtime. I tell everyone it was not just me. We were all in the right place at the right time.

First, Jim and his wife Nancy created The Charlie Foundation to Help Cure Pediatric Epilepsy. Next, the foundation funded five different workshops at Hopkins, where doctors, nurses and dietitians came to be trained. The foundation funded many more similar workshops after that. After being trained, the attendees would set up their own Ketogenic Diet programs at their own hospitals. And it continued from there. Many of those programs are doing well today. Some made changes to the diet, with disappointing results. The diet spread to Canada, was already in England, and now, more and more foreign countries are involved. It was a great honor to me to have been a guest at the first International Conference on the Ketogenic Diet held in Arizona in the spring of 2008, also funded by The Charlie Foundation.

Jim has never stopped. As a movie producer, he produced many videotapes for the doctors, dietitians and families, and other professionals—and was responsible for a second and third "Dateline" program. He also funded the book, *The Ketogenic Diet: A Treatment for Epilepsy*, which I coauthored with Dr. Freeman and his daughter Jennifer. The book is now in its fourth printing. (The first edition was funded by The Charlie Foundation.) Charlie's story was told in many popular magazines, including *Newsweek* and *People*. Jim has been a speaker at many fundraisers and Ketogenic Diet symposiums—and much, much more. He even produced a made-for-television movie, "First, Do No Harm," with Meryl Streep. It tells the true-life story about a former patient who had successfully started the diet at Hopkins. And I appeared in the movie as myself.

While all this was going on, and for several years afterward, we were accepting four to six patients nearly every week into the Ketogenic Diet program, allowing time off for vacations and holidays. As you can guess, it was very time-consuming, but also very rewarding. And the cooperation we received from the nurses, doctors and dietary personnel and other staff on the pediatric floors that housed these patients was heartwarming. They all wanted to help and were so excited when they saw that their patients' seizures had stopped, thanks to the diet.

By the end of 1994, we had started forty-one patients on the diet, and by the end of 1995, one hundred more. At the time this was happening, two fathers who were computer specialists designed a computer program, and our nurse, Jane Casey, started using this program in preparing the diet.

While we were at our busiest with so many patients, Dr. Janak Nathan came all the way from India, spending six to eight weeks in the clinic, learning every aspect of the Ketogenic Diet. When he returned to India, he started his own clinic, and taught the dietitians and nurses there how to do the calculations—the whole gamut. And his success has been outstanding. The diet works so well in India because they have a product there called ghee, made from drawn butter (butter with the water removed), making a more dense fat, which gives it much better ketogenic qualities. And ghee is very available in India. Money for medications is not an option there, so the diet is widely used. In India, many families are very poor, and Dr. Nathan, who has his own clinic, has yet to charge any patient who cannot afford to pay for his services. He is another "Tall Man."

Finally, in the fall of 1997, Dr. Freeman hired a full-time dietitian on his staff: Jane Spath. She and I worked together for about eight months. I retired in July 1998, pleased with my very able replacement.

Should the Ketogenic Diet be used as the first-line of treatment? My opinion is YES. You'll never know if you don't try it.

I'm proud to have been at Hopkins for most of fifty years, from 1948-1998 (with time off for the birth of my two children), and to have worked with the two most prominent doctors in the field of pediatric epilepsy. And I thank God for letting me be a part of The Charlie Foundation in perfecting and keeping the Ketogenic Diet alive.

I'd like to make one more point before closing: Some doctors say they are against children going on the diet because it is "unhealthy." When they say this, they are mainly referring to the fact that it is so high in fat. But our experience does not bear this out. First of all, in most cases, children go off the diet after two years, and can be on a regular diet for the rest of their lives. But there are cases where children have stayed on it much longer. When I am confronted with this objection to the diet, I like to give the example of Andrew Nealy. He was admitted to the Pediatric Unit at JHH in 1979 at the age of 12 to start the diet. Andrew was very disabled, and still is. His seizures were quickly controlled by the diet, and he is still on it today at age 43. He is still seizure-free. In some—very few—cases like these, people like Andrew have stayed on the diet for many years. But, the most interesting thing here is that Andrew, after thirty-one years on the diet, has extremely low cholesterol and triglycerides—after years of drinking two quarts of heavy cream a week for all this time!

In closing, I leave you with this thought: If you want to be successful, you must have a commitment and passion for what you are doing, have faith in yourself and be a little brave.

Milly has been given many honors in her life, but one that she still marvels at is being named an Alumna of the Year in the fall of 2009 by Mars Hill College, the junior college she attended before enrolling at the University of North Carolina. (Editor's note: In 1962, Mars Hill became a four-year college.) This, over sixty years after she graduated from college! (You may read the article about Milly in the Spring 2010 edition of the school's magazine at http://ftsmagazine.blogspot.com/2010/06/in-right-place-at-right-time.html.)

Please also watch this very touching video of Jim Abrahams' son Charlie, presenting an award to Milly in Phoenix, Arizona in April 2008 at the International Symposium on Diet Therapies. Go to http://charliefoundation.org/, and under the photo of Meryl Streep, click on "Charlie's Speech."

Beth Zupec-Kania, RD, CD:
Dietitian from 1993 to the Present

In my conversations with Jim, it became clear that he considers Beth Zupec-Kania to be as important in her own way to the success of the diet as Millicent Kelly has been in hers. Beth picked up where Milly left off. While the dietitians in Milly's day painstakingly crafted each child's diet by hand, Beth created a computerized program, which makes the job of creating individualized diets easier. She has trained other dietitians, and even parents, to prepare their children's meals more easily than was ever possible before. In addition to authoring several publications on the Ketogenic Diet, including a parents guide and professional manual, she's designed a web-based help line to support daily questions from dietitians. She also moderates a community forum for parents' concerns through The Charlie Foundation's website: http://charliefoundation.org.

In 1990, the year she started working at Children's Hospital of Wisconsin, Beth treated her first patient with the diet. She developed the Ketogenic Diet program there in 1993. In 2005, she began training personnel at other hospitals—physicians, nurses, hospitalists, pharmacists and dietitians. In 2006, she began working as the Director of Programs for The Charlie Foundation. In this capacity, she travels all around the world training dietitians and hospital staff to administer the Ketogenic Diet. She, too, is a tireless promoter of the diet and its benefits. (Editor's note: Hospitalists are practitioners, mainly physicians, but also nurse practitioners and physician assistants, who practice entirely in the hospital setting: http://www.hospitalmedicine.org.)

In Beth's words …

As Director of Programs for The Charlie Foundation, I do about fifteen trainings a year. I also get asked to go to other countries to train their staff. When I go abroad, I stay for a week and help them start a couple of patients on the diet, so that they become really comfortable with it. I've trained at least seventy centers so far, and have been to Saudi Arabia, Portugal, Germany and all over Canada. It is so interesting for me to go to these countries to see how they embrace the diet much more easily than it is embraced here in the United States.

I think Portugal is probably the country where interest in the diet took off the fastest. I'm not sure exactly why this is. It may be because it's a culture where they tend to see food as nourishment, as well as their medicine. It's a tiny country, and they're a little behind us in terms of commercialism. I visited in October

2007. Portugal has only six hospitals. All the neurologists came to my training and sent their staff, too. I trained them all together. We started two kids on the diet, and both of them benefited from it: One became seizure-free and the other had a 50 percent improvement. And both of these children were active and in regular classrooms. (http://honestmedicine.typepad.com/Keto%20News%20 Summer%202008.pdf)

I think there are a few reasons why the diet is embraced in other countries more readily than it is here. Probably most important, they don't have the array of seizure medications that we have. Either they don't have access to them, or their families can't afford them. But they can afford to do the diet therapy because the foods that are used on the Ketogenic Diet are available worldwide; they're basic foods, available in every culture.

Other reasons why US hospitals haven't embraced the Ketogenic Diet as widely and as readily as many other hospitals in countries around the world include: the pressure of pharmaceutical representatives, the apparent difficulty of administering the diet, and financial concerns.

In other countries, they don't have pharmaceutical representatives visiting doctors the way we do here. In fact, from what I can see, there is nothing like the US when it comes to sales calls to doctors from these reps, though that's starting to change. I've gone to Saudi Arabia three times. Doctors there have told me that they've felt the increased pressure from pharmaceutical companies in the past few years, whereas before, it was never an issue. But in most of the countries it isn't that way and they're more open to the diet.

Another problem with getting hospitals to use the diet is financial. Dietitians can't charge insurance companies for administering it. In fact, we can't charge for most dietary therapies, except for the three that we have federal legislation for: diabetes, and renal and cardiovascular diseases. At one time, I was reimbursed for administering the diet. But when our professional organization, the American Dietetic Association, lobbied for legislation to include reimbursement for these three specific diseases, they became the only kinds of nutritional counseling we could charge for. They were going for the big chronic diseases, where they'd get the most patients, and therefore, the most reimbursement.

So the fact that there is no reimbursement for the Ketogenic Diet is a major barrier to its implementation. The hospital just has to somehow absorb the cost; that's how my hospital functions. At the Children's Hospital of Wisconsin, we have a half-time dietitian dedicated to administering the diet. (I am a part-time employee there, as well, providing backup to the primary ketogenic dietitian.) The hospital gets no reimbursement for her time. The other half of her time she works as an inpatient dietitian, so she can charge for her work with hospitalized patients. My department traditionally is a money-losing department, just because we dietitians weren't smart ten years ago, and didn't demand reimbursement for any therapies other than those three. As new studies show disease improvement with this dietary therapy, we will go to the right people in Congress, who will hopefully support us. Then we will be able to add these other therapies for reimbursement. But as it stands now, the Ketogenic Diet is not one of those therapies.

A successful controlled randomized double-blind, Class 1 (i.e., "gold standard") study was recently conducted by Dr. Helen Cross in England. (http://www.medicalnewstoday.com/articles/106043. php) The results were very significant and very impressive. This study has put the diet on the map. It convinced many doctors that the success of the diet isn't just hearsay, or "anecdotal." It was all we needed for some doctors who had been skeptical before to say, "All right, we'll do this."

Another reason the diet hasn't become more widely used is that it requires mathematical calculations that are specific to each patient.

When Milly Kelly was doing the diet years ago, she and the other dietitians literally designed it "by hand." It was extremely rigid, and parents had to contact the dietitian whenever they needed anything changed. But I've designed a computer program, KetoCalculator, which is free to dietitians for calculating the necessary amounts of protein, carbohydrates and fats in the Ketogenic Diet: http://www. ketocalculator.com/ketocalc/. It takes the labor and the math mistakes out of the therapy. Today, it's used by hundreds of dietitians, and they can give access to it to the parents; parents can go in and create meals and snacks. When a program is designed for a child, we take into consideration their weight, their height and their activity level. Some kids need extra snacks on the days when they're more active, or the day after they've been more active. A parent might have a meal in mind for dinner and, at the last minute, realize she's short on avocado. She can open up her program and adjust her meal for less avocado. It just takes a few seconds to make this change with the KetoCalculator, and it makes the diet easier for the family.

We use the same program outside the United States, too, because it's Internet-based. I have people in Portugal putting foods in Portuguese into their database so the parents can have their meal plans printed in Portuguese instead of English. The database has every natural food available in the US. It includes creative recipes designed by parents that have been specially created for kids on the Ketogenic Diet. One of the first recipes I created was "keto mac and cheese," with heavy cream, cheddar cheese, and extremely low carbohydrate shirataki noodles that are mostly fiber. When you have all this blended together it tastes like real macaroni and cheese. (http://charliefoundation.org/recipes)

Things may be changing in our favor, at least in some areas. Until very recently (within the last six months of this writing), insurance companies were covering ACTH—a very expensive, side-effect-laden anti-seizure medication, a steroid—for a condition called infantile spasms. ACTH was, in fact, *the most expensive anti-seizure medication*, costing $8,000 a day—approximately $480,000 to $720,000 for two to three months, the average length of time babies had to stay on it. Both the Ketogenic Diet and ACTH have been found to be very effective in stopping infantile seizures. In fact, because of ACTH's side effects, the diet has been found to have similar efficacy with longer-lasting results. (Editor's note: There is more information about ACTH vs. the Ketogenic Diet in the Appendix, including links to comparative studies.) Yet, because insurance was covering it, more doctors were prescribing ACTH than the diet. Now, because of cost concerns, some insurance companies are no longer covering it, and the use of the Ketogenic Diet for infantile spasms has increased dramatically. An added benefit: The Ketogenic Diet is usually effective in two weeks for this epilepsy syndrome, while with most drugs, you have to wait two to three months for results.

There are several other conditions where the Ketogenic Diet is underutilized. For instance, there are children with a metabolic disorder called Glucose 1 Transporter Defect—Glut-1 Deficiency. (http://www.glut1.de/html-uk/index.htm) Some of these kids have seizures and some don't. We put them on the diet, and it can prevent them from being cognitively impaired—mentally retarded—because their brains, which can't use glucose, can use fat for energy instead. If you catch these kids early, when they're babies, you can actually prevent mental retardation. I'm working with five of these kids now, and they have all improved significantly with diet therapy. Since the diet is currently the only available therapy for this disorder, it is a lifelong treatment.

It has been published that the Ketogenic Diet is the only treatment that works with Glut-1. This disorder was described in the

1970s by Darrel DeVivo at Columbia University. He is the one who first wrote about it, and his protégé, a German doctor named Jeorg Klepper, is continuing the research, now that Dr. DeVivo is retired. (Dr. Klepper's website is http://www.glut1.de.) I was with him in England recently and he told me that he has just brought this therapy to the attention of some of the most knowledgeable neurologists in Germany, who are all sending him their patients who have Glut-1. As soon as you put these kids on the diet, it's amazing: their seizures dissipate, and they just perk up and do beautifully. The earlier they're diagnosed, the better. There are also other metabolic disorders—Pyruvate Dehydrogenase Deficiency and Glycogenosis Type V—for which the diet helps to improve cognition and control seizures, too. (For more about GLUT-1 Deficiency, see: http://www.hopkinsmedicine.org/neurology_neurosurgery/ specialty_areas/epilepsy/conditions/glut1_deficiency.html.)

There's another problem. Most children with epilepsy are being treated by pediatricians and neurologists. But it is *pediatric epileptologists* who know about all the treatments for pediatric epilepsy, including the Ketogenic Diet. The epileptologists, in my experience, have been the biggest champions of the diet. They are total believers. They see one child respond, and they realize that they've got to use the diet. Epileptologists are neurologists who have gone on for a fellowship to specialize in epilepsy. There are only four medically approved therapies that hospitals use to treat epilepsy: medications, the Ketogenic Diet, vagal nerve stimulation and surgery. In the US, there is a classification system for epilepsy centers. In order to be a level four Epilepsy Center (the highest level), you have to provide all four therapies.

Jim and I talk about the diet all the time. It's so wonderful. This is why I have such a passion for it. I can see what it does for kids. The problem is that people are waiting too long to start the therapy, and by the time so many of the kids are put on the diet—for instance, after the failure of five to seven anti-seizure medications—they already have severe disabilities. I'm passionate about getting as many children who need it on this diet.

Both Millicent Kelly and Beth Zupec-Kania have worked tirelessly to develop and promote the Ketogenic Diet. Their insight and hard work have helped thousands of children. Current and future dietitians would do well to learn from their example.

I want to thank both Milly and Beth for educating me and my readers. They've both been wonderful to work with.

Next, two more parents tell their stories.

First, Emma Williams.

CHAPTER 9

Emma Williams and Her Son, Matthew

Matthew's Friends—The Ketogenic Diet

When I initially told Jim Abrahams about my book, one of the first people he suggested I interview was Emma Williams, who lives in the United Kingdom. I can see why he did. In many ways, Emma's story is similar to that of so many parents of children with epilepsy. Like many of them, Emma was never told about the Ketogenic Diet by any of her son Matthew's doctors. Also, like many of them, when she found out about it on her own, through Jim Abrahams, and inquired about it, the doctors mocked her. When Emma was finally able to get Matthew on the diet, the changes he experienced were remarkable.

But Emma was not as lucky as Jim, in that much of the damage Matthew had endured from years of seizures, combined with the side effects of years of anti-convulsant medications, has been permanent. (Emma estimates that Matthew could have been saved nearly 25,000 seizures if he had been put on the diet when she first asked for it.) Still, she is grateful for the improvement that she feels her family has been blessed to have received from the diet.

Yet, Emma's anger at not having been allowed to try the diet earlier has propelled her to do amazing things, so that other parents won't have to suffer the way she did. Her story, like the others in this book, is inspirational.

Emma's story is a plea for the Ketogenic Diet to be offered to parents as one of the available options from the very beginning.

To see how remarkable Emma is, and how passionate about educating parents about the diet, be sure to watch this video: http://www.youtube.com/watch?v=T7DQOAeFFQo.

In Emma's words …

On September 8, 1994, my world changed forever with the birth of my son, Matthew. On that day, I learned how to feel total unselfish love and responsibility toward another human being.

Matthew weighed 9 lb., 14 oz. He was healthy and gorgeous, and everything was good in my world. Matthew was developing normally and I was busy going to all the mother-and-baby groups and being a competitive first-time mum. Matthew wasn't letting me down, either: We were winning all the development races in my group!

But that was all about to change—very dramatically and practically overnight.

When Matthew was 9 months old, his dad was giving him a bath when his first seizure occurred. I remember hearing Steve screaming downstairs for me to call an ambulance. I had never seen anything so frightening. This first seizure lasted for over fifteen minutes. While we waited for paramedics to arrive, I remember kneeling over Matthew and sponging him down with tepid water, praying to God not to let him die. I kind of kept it together until the paramedics got there. Once they arrived, I completely lost it.

In the hospital, we were told that it was probably a febrile convulsion, even though Matthew didn't have a fever. Maybe the bath water had been too hot? That was a guilt trip that Steve could have well done without, since there is no way he would have made that bath too hot; he was much too careful about those kinds of things.

It wouldn't take long for that theory to be blown out of the water. No pun intended.

Two weeks later, Matthew had another seizure. This one, in the middle of night, lasted over ten minutes. When the ambulance got to us, they administered Valium. This time in the hospital they said that although Matthew didn't have a fever, he must have a very delicate temperature gauge. In other words, he wouldn't necessarily have to have a high temperature in order to have a seizure, because it would probably be the speed at which his temperature rises that triggers the febrile convulsion. Or so they thought. Because of the length of the seizures, they decided to put him on Epilim, an anticonvulsant, "just until he grows out of having seizures." Chances are, they told me, by the time he reaches 5 years old, he won't have any more seizures. We were also given rectal Valium to administer, just in case he did have a seizure. We were told to take it everywhere with us.

We were also told that the meds would not have any side effects; Matthew would be fine. We could live with that. It wasn't ideal, but at least it wouldn't be this way forever, so we carried on with our plans to have another child. Soon I became pregnant with my Alice.

But the Epilim didn't stop Matthew's seizures. In fact, over the following six months, there were more and more seizures. Then, the dreaded status epilepticus—life-threatening prolonged and repeated seizures. Matthew was now constantly on medication and there were frequent "holidays" to various hospitals. I spent the vast majority of my pregnancy with Alice in the hospital with Matthew.

New words and phrases entered all my conversations: tonic clonic, MRI, EEG, complex partial, drops, sodium valproate, vigabatrin, topiramate, Valium, spasms, jerks. And "the favorite": epilepsy. My bedtime reading matter went from a good old trashy Jackie Collins book (no disrespect!) to *Your Child's Epilepsy: A Parent's*

Guide; *Epilepsy: the Facts*; *The Epilepsy Reference Book*; and *New Guide to Medicine and Drugs*—basically any book that had the word "epilepsy" in the title. I decided that, since knowledge is power, I would try to get as much knowledge as possible to try to understand what was happening to my son, and how I could help him the most.

By the time Matthew was 15 months old he was having seizures daily: tonic clonics, complex partials, absences and myoclonic jerks. He was formally diagnosed with "uncontrolled complex epilepsy." Only they couldn't tell me what had caused it; it was just "one of those things."

I was reading everything I could get my hands on about epilepsy, contacting every organization I could find, talking to whomever, wherever, to try and get answers and find information to help my boy. It was while I was on this quest that I first learned about the existence of the Ketogenic Diet. It seemed very promising to me.

When I asked Matthew's doctors about the diet, I was fobbed off and told that there was no real evidence that it worked and that it was very difficult to manage. Matthew was 2 years old when I first asked about the diet. Over the years I was denied the diet several times by our then-neurologist. She just wasn't interested in talking about the diet or even considering it. I was always told, "Drugs are the better option."

People are often surprised that I didn't take charge in these situations with Matthew's doctors, especially since I am so "feisty." They ask why I didn't just insist that Matthew be put on the diet. In retrospect, of course, I wish I had. I wish that nearly every day. But take charge with what? I had no energy left: I had to care for Matthew full time and, at the same time, look after his little sister. My marriage was breaking down, too. And there were the doctors to contend with, as well as social workers, educational psychologists, special needs schooling, friends and family, all of whom had their own opinions. Of course, there was always a mountain of paper-work to be completed, and reports to be written. All this was very overwhelming to someone who had never been through anything like this before, especially someone who had no support.

Besides all that, I kept telling myself that Matthew was be-ing taken care of at one of the best hospitals in the world. Great Ormond Street's reputation is well known. I reasoned that, if they didn't recommend the diet there, at such a pioneering hospital, then it must not work properly. I believed the neurologist when she told me how bad the diet was. I reasoned that she worked at Great Ormond Street, so she must know.

There's another thing, too: You don't want to upset the doctors. You are so frightened that they won't treat your child anymore if they get upset or angry with you. And some doctors can be very patronizing and treat you like a child yourself, when in fact you are a parent, who is terrified for your child.

I simply didn't know back then that Matthew just happened to have a neurologist who didn't believe in the diet. If we had been given a different neurologist, one who had a different opinion of the diet, even at the same hospital, things might have been very different. What it came down to then, and to a certain extent, what it can still come down to now, is whether or not your child's doctor believes the diet can help. Or, whether he or she believes that every possible drug combination has to be exhausted before any other treatment can be considered, especially a diet that is so high in fat, as the Ketogenic Diet is.

Even today, I still believe that Great Ormond Street Hospital is one of the best hospitals in the world. After all, it was there that, years later, I found Professor Helen Cross. And she now runs an excellent Ketogenic Diet Centre there.

So, the main reason I created Matthew's Friends was to empow-er parents so they wouldn't feel frightened or intimidated the way

I felt years ago, when speaking to their doctors about the Keto-genic Diet. I wanted to help parents so that they would be able to ask the relevant questions. And I wanted to dispel some of those myths about the diet that I had been told over the years. Most of all, through Matthew's Friends, I wanted to share my experience so that, years later, other parents won't have to feel the way I will have to feel every single day for the rest of my life: "If only I had fought harder and not taken no for an answer." People tell me all the time that I did the best I possibly could for Matthew with the information I had at the time. But, still, it doesn't ever stop the guilt for me. Every time my son has a seizure, there is always that small voice that says: "If only …"

Back then, we had a new baby, a diagnosis of uncontrolled complex epilepsy for our toddler, a huge mortgage, and no possibility of me going back to work because no one could care for Matthew. We were completely knackered (British for "exhausted").

By this time we were also finding out that AEDs (Anti-Epileptic Medication) did have serious side effects. Matthew's personality had totally changed. He would be very aggressive, biting and scratching everyone, knocking furniture over, trying to destroy anything he could get his hands on. You had to be very careful if he tried to cuddle you because the chances were that he was going in for a "bite" instead of a cuddle. We had to keep him away from his baby sister or supervise him very carefully around her. He would throw toys, scream all day at times, and wouldn't sleep at all. And some of these meds made the seizures worse. But when we went to the doctors and described all this, we were told that it wasn't the meds. They said that it was the "epilepsy developing," or that the side effects "would pass." Or that we needed to get him "up to the therapeutic dose," and then things would get better. We kept waiting and waiting for things to get better. But they never did.

We had to adjust rather rapidly to our new life—or rather, our "existence"—because that is how it felt: like an "existence." The awful thing was that at times I would be glad when Matthew had a seizure because at least he would sleep afterwards and things would be calm for a while. But then the guilt of feeling that way would totally consume me. I just felt a complete failure as a mother and was wracked with guilt at whatever choice I made and whatever I did. So many times I wanted to run as far away as possible and never see another seizure. But obviously I never could or would. My little Alice was my "angel child." She would cuddle me and play and remind me what it was like to be a "normal" mummy. Many a time that little girl kept me sane; she still does to this day!

Life was becoming more and more difficult for us as a family. We were frightened to take Matthew out in the summer in case he got too hot and had seizures. So, we locked ourselves up at home. And people avoided us, not knowing what to say and not wanting their children to see Matthew having a seizure. Some parents dragged their kids away from Matthew, frightened that their children might "catch" it. No more "mother and baby" groups for me, and no more the competitive mum. I just wanted Matthew to get through a day without injuring himself or others with his lashing out. His sister Alice described it this way, "My earliest memories of my brother aren't the best ones in the world. All I can remember is the constant shouting and him being so violent that you couldn't go near him without him either hitting or biting you." Naturally, I had to keep Alice away from him a lot of the time. Our home life was beginning to fall apart and the stress was unbearable. We had no support and didn't know what the hell to do next.

Everything was just a matter of muddling through.

Time was ticking by. Skills Matthew once had were fading fast and still no one could tell me why. When his seizures became uncontrollable by medication at home, we spent nights in the hospital in intensive care. Many episodes of status epilepticus occurred, which is a condition in which seizures occur non-stop, one after another. I don't think there's anything more frightening than the dreaded "status." Test after test continued to be carried out.

While all this was going on, the doctors were putting Matthew on all kinds of different drugs. Some made his fits worse; others made the fits slightly better—for a while. Some weeks he would be lying on the couch like a zombie, and other weeks, he would never sleep and spent all night shouting the house down. Years were spent getting up at 4 a.m., standing inside the playpen with the ironing board, while Matthew was wrecking the house outside the playpen! The only positive side of all this was that I never had a pile of ironing waiting to be done!

Matthew's seizure pattern changed over the years. Different types came along until Matthew had gone through the full spectrum. He went from seizing at any time to seizing mainly during sleep. It was extremely rare for anyone to have a full night's sleep in our house.

Matthew's mental age wasn't improving, either. Even though he was now 6 years old, cognitively and emotionally he was between 12 and 15 months old. He had no speech and was still in nappies (diapers). I was concerned; the school was concerned. There were no drugs left to try; every type of scan had been done on him; and he wasn't a candidate for surgery because they couldn't pinpoint which part of the brain the epilepsy was coming from. Besides, he now had so much scarring on his brain that it could have been the scarring that was causing a lot of the fits—although the fits were also causing scarring.

Matthew was now 6, and was under the care of Great Ormond Street Hospital. He had made no progress whatsoever. By this time I had seen Jim Abrahams' made-for-television film, "First Do No Harm," which is based on a true story about the Ketogenic Diet.

I could sympathize with so much of the story. It reminded me of what we had been through with Matthew. Still, whenever I spoke to the doctors about trying the diet, I was always given these same negatives:

    a. It was very difficult to manage.

    b. It was extremely unpleasant and unpalatable for the child. He could end up vomiting all the time.

    c. Although some success had been achieved with the diet, it was just not as effective as drugs, and it was a very "old fashioned" form of treatment.

    d. Considering that Matthew loved his food so much and was in good health otherwise, did I really want to put him through all that, for something that probably won't work anyway? "You have to think of his quality of life, Mrs. Williams!" Thanks. More guilt. Just what I needed.

The agencies involved with Matthew were now making noises that he might need to go into a residential home before too long, since he was a strong boy and getting so difficult to manage. The prospect of having to make that decision was breaking my heart: My boy was supposed to be at home with me and his sister, not anywhere else.

Doctors had told me that it was "unlikely" that Matthew would make "old bones" (old age), due to the number of seizures he was having. I was aware of the syndrome SUDEP (sudden unexpected death in people with epilepsy), which is similar to cot death. Unfortunately, Matthew fell into each and every one of the high-risk categories. I was told that if Matthew made it to the age of 12, then that would probably be the time when he would need to go into a residential home. It seemed like I was facing the option of Matthew going into a home or dying by the age of 12. It was heartbreaking.

Matthew was nearing 8, and his father and I had separated, pending divorce. The stress of the past few years finally took its toll on us. So now I was a single mum of two kids, one of whom was deteriorating at an alarming rate. At yet another appointment with Matthew's neurologist at Great Ormond Street, I again asked about the Ketogenic Diet.

This time was different. The doctor told me that her colleague, Professor Helen Cross, had recently started doing a clinical trial on the Ketogenic Diet. If I wanted, she would be happy to put Matthew's name forward for it. I practically bit her hand off saying yes! It was my last hope. There was absolutely nothing left to try and Matthew's epilepsy was worse than ever.

We made an appointment and I met with Professor Cross, Liz and Hannah (our "Keto Team"). They took me through the details about the trial, the diet, and of course, the paperwork. Even though I had wanted Matthew to try the diet for years, the prospect of actually doing it was daunting. I worried about how Matthew would cope with it. After all, my boy had an extremely healthy appetite and ate very well. Would not being able to have all his favorite things make him really miserable? Would he be hungry? How were his sister and I going to eat in front of him? Food was also a way I could nurture him and show him how much I loved him.

I worried about other restrictions it would create, too. For one thing, there would be no more school meals. And how would he be able to continue to go to respite care once a month? Respite care always provided such a welcome break for me. I was able to take Matthew there for one weekend a month. This gave me time to catch up on sleep, and also to have some time with Alice. It is so easy to forget how much fun it is being a mum when you have so much responsibility with a special needs child, especially one who needs constant supervision and care. When Matthew was at the respite centre, Alice and I would go out together for a movie and pizza. Or we would go swimming or to the park, all the "normal" kinds of things we couldn't do with Matthew. We would also just have a "girlie night" in front of the TV in our PJs; it was her chance to have her mum all to herself. I wondered what would happen if the respite centre wasn't prepared to take Matthew while he was on the diet. All these kinds of things went through my head.

Nevertheless, I still knew that whatever it took, we had to put Matthew on the diet. It had to be done. The diet was the only hope I had left.

Matthew could have started the diet in May 2002, but I held off for a couple of months. I cleared the decks at home. If I was going to do this, I was going to give it one hundred percent and I wasn't going to allow anything else to take up my time or energy. I also thought it best to start the diet when Matthew was with me all the time so I could keep a close eye on him.

The summer holidays began.

So did the Classical Ketogenic Diet!

I can only describe the first two weeks as a bloody nightmare. For one thing, it seemed as if I was spending all day every day in the kitchen preparing Matthew's meals. I weighed and then reweighed his food to make sure it was right. Because his meals contained so much fat, they were tiny in comparison to what he had been eating before. It took a while to get my head around the fact that he was still taking in the same number of calories as before. Because of the different proportions of fat, carbs and protein, there was less actual food on his plate. He was grumpy and miserable. He spent most of the time shouting and seemed extremely unhappy. He was still having seizures, so he was either shaking or shouting. The guilt I was feeling was terrible. His sister and I didn't eat in front of him. We were reduced to eating the odd bar of chocolate while sitting on the toilet.

After the first three to four days, Matthew started to calm down. Over the next few days, he calmed down even more, so much so that he just lay on the settee. He was eating the meals I prepared for him, but the dirty looks I was getting from him were something to behold.

I was still living in the kitchen in between dealing with Matthew's seizures and being on the phone with either Liz or Hannah at Great Ormond Street. I must have driven them mad! The problem was that Matthew had calmed down so much by now that I was having problems waking him up. He had stopped drinking and was becoming dehydrated, so I was syringing fluids into him as much as I could. But it wasn't enough. Matthew had now gone into what is known as excess ketosis and metabolic acidosis. While ketosis, carefully monitored while a child is on the diet, is not dangerous, excess ketosis and metabolic acidosis are. The side effects are drowsiness, a flushed face, and in some cases, panting breath. Matthew's breath also stank of pear drops, or "ketone breath," as we came to know it. I knew he was in trouble. On advice from Hannah during what must have been my tenth phone call with her that day, I called an ambulance. The blue lights appeared and the entire neighborhood came out to wave us off.

On the way to the hospital, the paramedics gave Matthew some oxygen, which seemed to perk him up a bit. Once at the hospital, the pediatrician came to see him. I went through the details and told him that Matthew was on the Ketogenic Diet, to which I got the response, "The what diet?" This was a response that I have now grown accustomed to.

While we were waiting in A&E (Accident and Emergency, which is the same as the ER, or the emergency room in the United States), Matthew decided he was thirsty and proceeded to drink a very large cup of his juice and then another! The upshot was that he was as bright as a button fifteen minutes later and no longer needed an IV. After all, he had had a good long sleep during the day, a ride in an ambulance with blue flashing lights and sirens going, a good whiff of oxygen and a couple of large cups of juice. I think it's called "little boy heaven." I, on the other hand, had reached the "lost the plot" stage and was eyeing his rectal Valium longingly. The only thing that stopped me using the stuff was where I would have to shove it.

My mother collected her lively, bouncing, smiling grandson and her "heap" of a daughter from the hospital and took us home.

I got up the next morning and braced myself for the new day. I wondered what it would have in store for us. My lively, bouncing, smiling son also got up and he stayed that way all day. The only thing that wasn't "right" about Matthew that day was his seizures: He didn't have any!

He didn't have any the following day either, or the one after that. I got to the point where I was almost frightened to breathe, just in case it set him off again. I couldn't believe what I was seeing.

Matthew ate all his meals. He was happy and calm. He was sleeping well and waking at a more reasonable hour. Instead of the 4 a.m. I had grown used to over the years, he was now waking up at about 6:30 a.m. The first time he slept later I remember waking up and running, screaming his name, from my bedroom to his, fearing that he had become a victim of SUDEP—that I was going to find my child dead in his bed. But on the contrary, he was sound asleep, or rather, he was—until I had woken him with my scream-ing and bursting into his room. His face was a picture: Let's just say that he was not impressed that I had woken him up. I, on the other hand, was so relieved that I thought I was going to vomit. Anyway, it didn't take me long to get used to this far more dignified time of getting up in the morning. Matthew didn't have a single seizure for nearly two weeks. Then he had one tonic clonic and that was it for another couple of days. Then he had a couple of absences and that was it for a few more days.

My time in the kitchen was now greatly reduced, too. I had got to grips with the diet and had got myself organized. Vegetables were steamed and batched; meat was weighed and batched, as were puddings. Spare ketogenic meals such as quiches were made and frozen in case of emergency or a sudden packed lunch being needed.

Matthew went back to school and every day, his lunch went with him. He went to respite too. I prepared a file which contained copies of all the information on the Ketogenic Diet, a shopping list, helpful hints to make things easier while managing the diet, and meal plans where I had worked out all the weights of everything for his meals. As long as the respite centre followed my meal plans to the letter, there would be no problem with Matthew's diet. They were more than willing to do this, and before Matthew went, I visited the centre and went through everything with them. I gave them all the details and the information that they needed. They were great.

After a very shaky start culminating in that one hospital visit, we have never looked back. From having between ten and twenty seizures per day, Matthew now has, on average, three per week. Some weeks, he has none at all; other weeks, slightly more. But we have never gone back to the amount he used to have when he was just on medication.

Speaking of medication, Matthew had been on a huge amount: 600 mg of gabapentin (Neurontin) per day and 200 mg of topiramate (Topomax) per day. He would also have clobazam at times if he was having a particularly rough patch; or he would have clonazapam. He would also need rectal Valium at frequent times, too, and I would carry paraldehyde everywhere with us if the rectal Valium didn't work.

Now Matthew was on no medications. All medications had been thrown in the bin. The only thing I kept in the fridge was rectal Valium, just in case. And occasionally I had to use it. Normally, this would happen when Matthew was building for a change in his diet following a growth spurt, or when he was not very well. But again, it was nowhere near the amount it used to be.

After a few months on the diet, Matthew called me "Mum" for the very first time. I didn't stop blubbing for about four days. No money in the world can buy that feeling. Now, when he comes home on his school bus and sees me coming to get him, he says, "Mum Mum." I feel like I win the lottery every day.

Matthew made more progress at school in the first six months of being on the diet than he had in the previous six years. Of course, they were delighted with him. All talk of Matthew going into a residential home also stopped. No need. My boy is staying at home with his sister and me.

There have been rough patches on the diet when his seizures have increased. As I mentioned earlier, when Matthew was experiencing a growth spurt, the diet had to be adjusted. And when he is unwell, too. But the rough patches we have now are nowhere near as bad as they used to be before going on the diet.

For me, the diet meant that I always had to be organized as far as food was concerned. I had to make sure that I had everything I needed. I could never take a day off from the diet and I couldn't just hand it over to someone else and say "get on with it"—unless, of course, I had trained them first. But, thankfully, Matthew has an excellent godmother who would help, as well as a first-class caretaker. Funnily enough, she is also called Emma.

When Matthew was on the diet, I always had to be vigilant that he ate only the foods that were on the diet—and in the correct amounts. At times, I felt like I was the only mother in the world who told other children not to share their treats with her child, although I have to say that Matthew did not even try to eat any other food. It is like he knew that what he ate was helping him and making him feel better.

While Matthew was on the diet, we tried to do everything any other family would do. He had a birthday party like any other child, and I had all the family around. Out of respect for Matthew, we all ate ketogenic food: I made sugar-free jellies, peanut butter sandwiches (using lettuce instead of bread), dips and—of course—birthday cake. (Yes, a ketogenic chocolate cake can be done!) Matthew had a great time and so did we. On his second year of the diet, I got a lot braver and actually threw him a trampolining birthday party with all his friends from school. Foodwise, it was easy. I did a "boxed" party tea. Every child got a fancy box (similar to a McDonald's Happy Meal® box) and I put everyone's food in their box. Matthew had the same box but with his own food in it, which was so much easier because all his food had been weighed out beforehand. I gave the partygoers a proper chocolate cake to take home with them, whereas Matthew had his keto chocolate cake.

We would sometimes go and stay with friends and family for weekends. When we went out to eat, I would phone the restaurant first and explain our situation; I'd take Matthew's food in with me and they would heat it up for him. If any restaurant refused to do this, then obviously we didn't eat there. (And I would then phone the local paper and completely trash them! What can I say? I get annoyed with small-mindedness.)

I am not an unrealistic person, I know that this diet will not work for every child who has epilepsy, but it does work for many children. And it is certainly worth a try. There is nothing to lose and everything to gain.

I'd like to dispel the most commonly cited negatives doctors use when they are trying to discourage parents from putting children on the diet:

> a. The diet does not have to be difficult to manage. It can be daunting at first, but it doesn't take long to get into the swing of things. Once your confidence

builds, it is about as difficult/time-consuming as making up babies' bottles once a day.

b. Unpleasant and unpalatable. It can be if you just swamp everything in double cream, but it really doesn't have to be. There are loads of recipes/ideas that can make lovely meals that your child can enjoy. And you don't have to be a chef to be able to make them. But we have a chef here at Matthew's Friends, if you need one.

c. Old-fashioned and not effective. The diet may be considered "old-fashioned," but it works. As for not being effective, it won't be for every child, but then again, neither are the drugs. But it is effective for many, and I will happily argue until I am blue in the face with anyone who tries to tell me any different!

d. Quality of life. Matthew has the best quality of life he has ever had. And now, thanks to the Ketogenic Diet, we do, too.

By 2005, Matthew had been on the Ketogenic Diet for nearly four years and he was coming up to 12 years old. Because of puberty and a really restrictive amount of carbs, his dietitian and I decided to change him from the classical version of the diet to the MCT (medium chain triglyceride) version, which is a little easier to do. On it, he was allowed a lot more food. He couldn't believe his eyes (or his luck) when he had his first meal that contained chips! (For a discussion of the differences between the regular and the MCT versions of the diet, see http://site.matthewsfriends.org/uploads/pdf/TypesofKetoDiet.pdf.)

Some children need only be on the diet for a couple of years and can then be weaned off and their seizures will never return. Matthew has never been completely seizure-free. But that was never my aim, since I knew how brain damaged he was. Obviously, there is always the hope that your child will be seizure-free and stay that way forever, but I knew that the chances of Matthew ever being that way were extremely small. He had massive amounts of scarring on his brain. He was still a baby mentally. So I knew that he was never going to catch up. I knew the seizures and all the meds had taken their toll on my son, but I just wanted him to have the best quality of life he could have. And he certainly got that. After two years, most children are able to be weaned off the diet. But I wasn't emotionally able to do this. The reason, plain and simple, was fear. I was terrified that if I weaned him off, the seizures would come back. And there was no way I could face going back to how things were. Besides, he was healthy and happy. The MCT diet was a lot easier for us, so there was no need to wean him off.

But after another two years on the MCT version of the Ketogenic Diet, I decided to try and wean Matthew off the diet completely, with the understanding that if things got a lot worse, we could put him straight back on. Professor Cross and I made a plan for him and I started to wean. The diet had affected Matthew's growth, but we weren't too worried about that. He was doing okay, so having to sacrifice a few centimeters of growth didn't seem too much of a hardship. We also thought that we would give his body a bit of a break from ketosis and see what would happen. Once again, fear was overtaking me. But we had to try.

We weaned Matthew off the diet, but I still didn't go mad with the carbs. We just added a bit each week and reduced the amount of MCT oil that he had to have with the diet until eventually he wasn't having any additional fat in his diet. He did fine and nothing major happened, apart from the fact that once off the diet, Matthew grew like a weed. He shot up in height and quickly made up for all the "reduced" growth he had on the diet.

Over the next few months I noticed that his seizures weren't increasing in number, but they did increase in length of time—not to a dangerous level, but they were lasting about two minutes. I wasn't happy about this. I again talked things over with Professor Cross. As most of Matthew's seizures were at night, we agreed to carry on with his "keto break" for a year, and put him on a little bit of valproate (Epilim/Depakote) to see if it would bring the length of time down. If I noticed any adverse reactions to this, I could stop the medication and we would have a rethink.

Matthew started on a really small dose of Epilim, and it did help reduce the length of time of his seizures. We didn't notice any side effects from the med. I could live with that, although putting him back on a med felt like we were taking ten steps back. It felt awful at the time, a bit like failing. But that was not the case. It was doing what was best for Matthew and giving him the best quality of life. Because now I finally had a neurologist, Professor Helen Cross, with whom I could discuss my worries and fears, someone who would listen and work with me, I felt far more in control and confident about our future. Besides, this was just a "keto break." I would be taking Matthew off meds in a year and putting him back on the diet.

JANUARY 2010

We are still on that keto break!

Matthew is still on his really small dose of Epilim (not even classed as "therapeutic") and doesn't need anything else. We can live with that. But always at the back of my mind I have these diets to fall back on in case things get worse again.

I also finally got a proper diagnosis for Matthew: He has Dravet Syndrome, which is a severe form of epilepsy; the gene mutation has been confirmed. (For a definition, go to: http://www.ninds.nih.gov/disorders/dravet_syndrome/dravet_syndrome.htm.) After all those years of searching, it wasn't until Matthew was 14 years old that we finally got the answer. Now I understand why some of the drugs reacted so badly with him. It was because there are certain medications children with Dravet should not be given, medications that can make these children worse. And boy, did they ever make Matthew worse! I had such mixed emotions when I finally got the diagnosis: I was glad that I finally had an answer that would make Matthew's treatment a lot clearer, since we now knew which drugs to avoid. But I also had to deal with a very unclear future for Matthew, since Dravet Syndrome is a complicated condition. However, the diet is known to work very well for Dravet children, which is probably one of the reasons Matthew responded so well to it. But once I found out that he had Dravet Syndrome, I felt even more guilty for not pushing harder for the diet in the first place.

The big thing I have to deal with now is that Alice has to be tested for the Dravet gene. It is like this nightmare never ends. The thought that Alice could possibly have a child like Matthew (however small that risk might be) frightens me. Don't get me wrong, I wouldn't want to be without Matthew. He has taught me so much and I am extremely blessed to have him. And I feel honored that I am the one taking care of this beautiful boy. But there has been a lot of heartache along the way and there will be more to come. As a mother, I don't want to see my girl having to go through any of what I have gone through.

Matthew's seizures are still small by comparison to pre-diet days, about 70 to 80 percent reduced. They are not very long and occur mostly at night. The sad thing is that over the past couple of years, Matthew has lost his ability to walk. This doesn't happen to every Dravet kid, but their walking can be affected this way. And the fact that Matthew had so much brain damage due to all the earlier seizures and medications has obviously not helped the situation. There is now no question that Matthew would have always been disabled and had seizures, but he could have been a lot better than he is now, if we had found the diet earlier. And he might not have ended up in a wheelchair. He could have been just a few years behind his "real" age, instead of having a mental age of about a 12- to 15-month-old child (although he understands far more than you think!). He can do a mean crawl around the house. We have a big fancy wheelchair now with a motor attached to it—it saves my back! Alice and Matthew have great fun whizzing around the shopping malls.

It is the care side of Matthew that takes the time now and is the biggest factor in our lives—not the seizures—a massive turnaround from pre-keto days. Matthew no longer goes away to respite, as he is happiest at home. So his fantastic carer, Emma, who is still with us, comes in and looks after him when I am away on Matthew's Friends business and they have a great time.

Matthew turned 16 this September 2010. He is nearly six feet tall and is as strong as an ox. This is a massive achievement for a boy who had years of devastating seizures and who was written off by professionals at one point as being deemed either dead or in a residential home by the age of 12.

We are celebrating big-time this year and there is not a day that goes past when I don't thank God for this diet. It saved this family and gave my son the best quality of life he has ever had.

But I don't think I will ever be able to forgive myself and Matthew's doctors for the fact that we had to wait so long for the Ketogenic Diet. Matthew was 9 months old when he started having seizures. He was 2 years old when I first asked his doctors about the diet. They not only talked me out of it; it felt like they were almost laughing at me for even wanting to try it. I was made to feel like some kind of bad mother because I wanted to subject my child to this diet. It wasn't until Matthew was almost 8, in 2002, that Matthew was finally put on the diet. By that time, he had experienced tens of thousands of seizures, and had been taking a cocktail of anti-seizure drugs, which didn't stop his seizures. Matthew incurred irreversible brain damage from the combination of those nearly six years of seizures and from the side effects from so many drugs. All of this has affected Matthew's development and his quality of life. The Ketogenic Diet offered Matthew another choice. I wish we had been encouraged to take advantage of that choice six years earlier. I wish I had been able to push harder for it.

I couldn't (and still can't) get it out of my head that, had we not been discouraged from trying the Ketogenic Diet in 1996, when I first asked his neurologist about it, Matthew would be a very different boy today. We would have been able to avoid all those years of seizures and medications. And today, I have no doubt that Matthew would have made so much more progress than he has been able to make. I really don't believe he would have had to be in a wheelchair permanently. And I know that we could have gotten more speech from him and better communication skills. I am very grateful for the quality of life we have now, compared to how bad it was before the diet. Still, it is just too distressing to even think about "what could have been"—if we had only started the diet years earlier.

But still, I am very grateful that things did eventually get better for Matthew and for us, thanks to the diet. In 2004, I created Matthew's Friends: www.matthewsfriends.org. I am proud to say that we work side by side with The Charlie Foundation, set up by Jim Abrahams, to spread the word about the diet throughout the world. The goal of both organizations is that, very soon, parents throughout the world won't have to be without knowledge of the diet, like we were, when we first consulted neurologists for our children.

Even today, some neurologists will still try to push massive amounts of drugs on children, even after the first two drugs fail. This is particularly maddening to both Jim and me, since it is well known throughout the medical profession and the epilepsy organizations that if the first two anti-epileptic medications don't work, then the chance of any other epilepsy drug working is reduced to about 10 percent. This is why Matthew's Friends advocates that the diet be made available as a treatment after two anti-epileptic medicines have been tried. This falls in line with the recently published 2008 Consensus Statement made by some of the world's leading medical professionals using the diet: http://www.epilepsy.com/ epilepsy/keto_news_mar09. Personally, I believe that parents should be told about the diet from the very beginning, when a child first starts having seizures. It is an extremely valuable option, and should be presented as such.

Matthew's Friends will not stop until every parent who wants the Ketogenic Diet for his or her child is able to get it, and with it, an opportunity for a chance at a better life.

In October 2010, Emma and Matthew's Friends hosted the International Symposium on the Dietary Treatments for Epilepsy and Other Neurological Disorders in Edinburgh, Scotland. There were scientific presentations for professionals, including neurologists, epileptologists, research scientists, nurses, dietitians and other allied health professionals. There were also programs for families. To learn more about the work being done by Matthew's Friends, see the Appendix and http://site.matthewsfriends.org/.

CHAPTER 10

Jean and Julie McCawley

A Mother and Daughter with Two Causes

Of all the stories in this book, Jean McCawley's is the most complicated. Most of the advocates who have contributed chapters have one main mission: to get the word out about the little-known treatment that saved their own, or their child's, life. Jean has two missions: the first, to educate people about Stevens Johnson Syndrome (SJS), the condition that almost killed her infant daughter, Julie, in 1994. Because of SJS, Julie now has several "side-effects" that complicate her life. If Jean had been told about the Ketogenic Diet before Julie had been given Phenobarbital, Julie would not have almost died, and she would not be nearly blind today. She would have been able to live a completely normal life. But Jean was not told about the diet. She didn't find out about it until she saw Jim Abrahams on "Dateline NBC." So, her second (and equally important) mission is to educate people about the diet. Julie, now 16 years old, has become equally vocal about getting the word out, as you will see from this chapter. I think you'll be impressed by both Jean and Julie.

In Jean's words ...

~

If I had been told about the Ketogenic Diet back in 1994 when my 10-month-old daughter Julie had her first grand mal seizure, our lives would have been very different. I would have chosen the diet over drugs, and she would have recovered from her epilepsy.

And that would have been that. We would have been saved many years of avoidable suffering and tragedy.

But that's not the way it happened for us, which is why I want everyone to know our story: so that more parents will learn about the diet as a first-line therapy, rather than a last—barely whispered, almost-by-accident—resort.

For her first ten months, Julie was a perfectly normal baby. Even as a newborn, she was more alert than most babies. At 2 weeks of age, people thought she was 6 weeks old! By the time she was 6 months old, she was crawling and even babbling, trying to say words. By 11 months of age, she had a thirty-word vocabulary. Except for one ear infection, Julie was an extremely healthy, happy baby.

So, nothing could have prepared me for her first seizure. I remember it as if it were yesterday: I was getting ready for work. I'd fixed bottles for Julie and for my 20-month-old niece, Kathleen. (My sister Leslie and her children lived with me and our mom at the time.) Both babies were in the crib. I had just taken a shower and was drying my hair. I was standing before the mirror at my dresser, when I had a horrible feeling that "something" was wrong. I ran over to the crib. Kathleen looked fine, but Julie's eyes were wide open, and she was staring at the wall. I picked her up. She was stiff as a board and white as a ghost. Having never actually seen a dead person before—and having never seen a seizure, either—I thought Julie was dead. Luckily, my sister had taken Infant CPR classes, so she started doing CPR on her, and Julie started to shake. My sister said, "She's okay; she's having a seizure." My mother called 911.

At the hospital, the doctor prescribed the anti-seizure drug Phenobarbital. When I asked what the side effects were, I was told there was only one: drowsiness.

I was not prepared for what lay ahead. I was totally unaware that something as simple as a tiny pill would begin a lifetime nightmare for us.

For two weeks, drowsiness was Julie's only side effect. And of course, we were grateful she wasn't having seizures. Then, one morning when she got up, her right eye was swollen shut. By evening, her other eye was swelling. I couldn't figure out what was going on. I kept checking to see if there was something in her eyes. There wasn't. I rocked her all night.

When Julie developed a high fever, I took her to the pediatrician. While we were there, she began developing blisters across her shoulders and on her mouth. It was awful. The pediatrician diagnosed her with chicken pox, conjunctivitis, a double ear infection and strep throat. This seemed very strange to me, since she hadn't been exposed to any of these illnesses. And her blisters were so huge that I remember thinking, "If this is chicken pox, it is the most horrifying case I've ever seen."

Julie's condition continued to worsen as the day went on. She could no longer drink out of a bottle, because her mouth and throat were filled with blisters. And she continued to run a high fever. I worried that since she was not taking any liquids, she would become dehydrated. I called the hospital and was told to wait another six hours and if she still didn't have a wet diaper by then, to bring her in.

When I took her to the emergency room she was very dehydrated, so they started an IV. They gave her the missed dose of Phenobarbital from the night before, another dose that night and another the next day. This went on for four days. But Julie wasn't getting any better. In fact, she was getting progressively worse. Her lungs were collapsing. And her blisters continued to grow to the size of half dollars. And they were breaking open. Soon her skin was coming off in sheets, and her face was unrecognizable. She looked like she had been deep fried.

Still, the doctors continued to call it "chicken pox." They said it was just a very serious case. They said the reason she looked so bad was because she had to have been exposed to the disease over a long period of time. I told them that Julie hadn't been exposed to anyone with chicken pox. They told me I must have been mistaken, that Kathleen might have had a very mild case, so mild that no one knew she had it. So that even if we hadn't known Kathleen had chicken pox, she could have infected Julie. I knew this wasn't so.

This was the first time that doctors told me that they understood my child better than I did. There were to be many other similar times over the years.

Four days later, thanks to a nurse who had seen Stevens Johnson Syndrome (SJS) before, we got a diagnosis. Julie had SJS, resulting from the side effects of Phenobarbital. I remember how happy I was at the time, thinking: "Finally, we know what is wrong. Now she can get better." Then a doctor told me, "Jean, this is not a good thing." That was August 18, 1994.

As I was to find out, Stevens Johnson Syndrome is far from a good thing. It is one of the most severe adverse reactions to a medication that a person can suffer from. And anti-convulsants are among the top causes. (Other medications that can trigger SJS are over-the-counter medications like ibuprofen. The worst offender is the sulfa drug, Bactrim. The worst anti-seizure drug is lamotrigine, or Lamictal.)

Julie got worse and worse, and quickly escalated to Toxic Epidermal Necrolysis (TEN), which is the most severe form of SJS. For twenty-seven days, she was treated in the hospital's burn unit with burns over 80 percent of her body. Julie's skin was debrided every day. This means that, every day, they put her in a big silver pan, filled with warm water with a capful of bleach to kill any bacteria. They put gauze in the water and used it to scrape off her dead skin. By the time they had debrided her, the pan was filled with dead skin and blood. Afterwards, they wrapped her whole body in bandages. Watching the process was terrifying. Julie was on morphine for the pain and had a feeding tube for nutrition.

Over the years, Julie has suffered terribly. She didn't hear until she was 18 months old, because the blisters in her ears had ruptured and wept over her eardrums. The blisters had to be removed by an ear, nose and throat doctor. I watched in horror as doctors performed traumatic procedures on her eyes to save her sight. On her first birthday, I was told my baby would go blind.

Many of the ravages of Stevens Johnson Syndrome have been permanent. Her eyes, ears and throat suffered extensive damage. She is blind in her right eye and has low vision in her left. She has photophobia (inability to tolerate bright lights), dry eye syndrome, a swallowing disorder, and scarring in her esophagus and inside her ears. Since the light hurts her eyes, when she goes outdoors, she needs someone to walk with her, and she has to wear a hat and sunglasses, and use a cane.

And Julie is one of the lucky ones. Many SJS patients die.

Even though every doctor who came in contact with us knew that Phenobarbital had caused all of Julie's troubles, at no time were we offered the Ketogenic Diet. The neurologists must have known that the diet had been used successfully at Johns Hopkins since the 1920s, because it had been written about in their journals. Yet not one doctor even mentioned the diet to us. As a matter of fact, as soon as she was released from the hospital, I was advised to put her on drugs again. Dilantin and something else. But by now, I was terrified of these drugs. I refused, even though Julie continued to have seizures.

It was after our horrible month in the hospital with SJS that Jim and Charlie Abrahams' story appeared on "Dateline." (http://www.youtube.com/watch?v=STPOEFfQdjw) If it hadn't been for Jim, I don't know what I would have done. As I watched the program, I just knew that the Ketogenic Diet would be our answer. At the end of the show, they gave an address for The Charlie Foundation. I wrote Jim a letter, and told him all about Julie and what we had been through. I didn't expect to hear from him, but I did. I was at work, and I got a call from my mom, who was taking care of Julie. She told me that Jim, Charlie's dad, had called.

I don't think I can describe in words how I felt that this wonderful man would go out of his way for us, a single mom in Colorado, and her baby. What a wonderful, caring human being. I was touched and amazed. I called Jim back. He told me all about the diet, and said I should talk to the doctors about getting Julie on it. So I started talking to doctors and right away, a wall went up. "No, Jean, the diet won't work. We need to give her another drug." I told them that, no matter what, I wanted Julie on this diet. But I had an HMO, and I knew I'd have to fight to get her on the diet.

Over Thanksgiving that year, Julie had seventeen seizures. The seizures were so bad that she had to be taken by ambulance to the hospital. I think I wore the doctors down, because this time, they actually asked me what I wanted to do. Again, I said, "I want her on the Ketogenic Diet." They must have finally realized that I just didn't want her on drugs. I was terrified of pharmaceutical options: Even Depakote, the drug they put her on previously to break her status epilepticus, hadn't worked. This time, the neurologist said, "Okay, we'll do it." And they tried her on the MCT oil diet, which looked like formula in a bottle. (http://www.epilepsy.com/epilepsy/keto_news_august07) It had all the high fat in it, like the regular Ketogenic Diet. They had her fasting, and Jim would call me the whole time, checking on how Julie was doing, on how it was going.

Unfortunately, because they didn't really know how to administer the diet in this hospital, they made a terrible mistake. The nurse read the order wrong. She thought that the meal they had sent up for Julie was for the whole day, when in fact it was only for one meal. So she watered that meal down to one-third, and Julie's blood sugar went down to an extremely low level. Julie went into status epilepticus, which means that her seizures were practically non-stop. Julie had forty-four grand mal seizures in less than twenty-four hours, and the shortest one lasted for twenty minutes. The longest: fifty minutes. The seizures caused her heart to stop; she went into cardiac arrest. They loaded her with the maximum loading dose of Depakote, an anti-seizure medication, and they gave her so much Ativan that she became comatose. This time, when Jim called, he was told that Julie was in the ICU, in a coma. He was furious, and contacted Dr. Freeman at Hopkins. Jim told me that Dr. Freeman called the hospital and said, "If you don't know what you're doing, then don't do it!"

Meanwhile, Julie's prognosis was looking even grimmer. The neurologists told me that she would never walk. They said she'd probably never do much of anything, because her brain had been fried from so many seizures.

I wanted desperately to take Julie to Hopkins. I knew that the Ketogenic Diet, properly administered, was the only thing that would save her.

The way we finally got the diet done right is quite a story.

A local radio show in nearby Denver held a contest called "The Twelve Days of Christmas." My sister Leslie wrote a letter to the station. She said that her wish was for her niece Julie to be put on the Ketogenic Diet. She wrote about Julie and all we had been through, and she wrote about the diet: that it is a cure for epilepsy, and that they do it at Johns Hopkins. In her letter, she wrote that we just needed to find a way to get the diet done correctly.

My sister's letter won as "Christmas Wish #11." This was all a complete shock to me. I didn't even know she had entered the contest. The station called me while I was at work. I cry today as I remember it. They said they had my sister's letter in front of them. And they said they had Diana Pillas on the line. Diana, who died very recently, was the wonderful nurse from Johns Hopkins, who used to work with Millicent Kelly, the dietitian who championed the diet for over fifty years. The show host read my sister's letter, and then, Diana Pillas came on the phone and told me that she, and "the team at Hopkins," were going to do everything they could to help us to get the diet administered in Denver. They had found us a doctor in Denver, who had worked with Mrs. Kelly, to help us.

You may listen to this wonderful audio of the radio show, with Leslie, Diana Pillas and me. (I'm the one who is crying throughout the whole segment.) The video is accompanied by a wonderful slide presentation, so that you can see actual photos of Julie throughout the years: http://www.youtube.com/watch?v=2zUM5CsObsQ.

We started Julie on the Ketogenic Diet in Denver. But, remember, I still had the HMO. Unfortunately, they wouldn't let the pediatrician who had worked with Mrs. Kelly, Dr. Edra Weiss, help us with the diet. But Dr. Weiss and I did meet. One day, she was visiting another patient, another baby who happened to be in the same hospital room as Julie. She looked at Julie's chart, realized who we were, and crossed the room to me. She said, "I just want to tell you something, Jean. Your HMO doesn't want my help. They won't let me work with you on the diet. But they're not going to mess it up, because, this time, the whole world is watching. And they know it."

On December 26, 1994, Julie went on the diet, and that was the end of her seizures. Two-and-a-half years later, she had her first ice cream cone. We all stood around watching her. My sister's mother-in-law was a nervous wreck. She kept saying, "Don't let her have it. She'll have a seizure."

But I said, "There's a time when we have to say, 'Let's see how she does. Let's let her be a kid. Let's watch.'" That's what we did.

And Julie never seized again. Ever.

So now I have two causes. One, of course, is getting the Ketogenic Diet known to every parent whose child is diagnosed with epilepsy, before they are started on these dangerous anti-seizure drugs. It is so important that parents be given a choice, so that they don't have to stumble on the diet on their own. Jim Abrahams has been such a help to us that Julie and I want to support him in any way that we can. That's why Julie spoke at The Charlie Foundation conference, "Dietitians and Nurses Forum: Dietary Therapies for Epilepsy," in November 2009. She also sang beautifully. And that's why I am so happy to be part of this book. (Editor's note: For Julie's presentation at the November 2009 conference, go to http://charliefoundation.org/ and click on the thumbnail titled "Julie's Story," directly under the photo of Meryl Streep.)

Our other cause is a foundation, which we started in March 1996. We first called it The Julie Foundation for Allergic Drug Reactions. It is now called The Stevens Johnson Syndrome Foundation: http://sjsupport.org/. It's a nonprofit organization whose mission it is to provide people with the information that we struggled so hard to find. Adverse Drug Reactions are the fourth leading cause of death in the United States, yet fewer than one percent of these reactions are reported to the FDA. This has to change. We are also working on getting more medical research into Stevens Johnson Syndrome and Toxic Epidermal Necrolysis (SJS/TEN).

When Julie was first diagnosed with epilepsy in 1994, I was told we would never hear of another person with SJS. We have reached around the world with our SJS Support Group and have received hundreds of requests. We have sent out hundreds of packets with information that was not readily available to us when Julie was diagnosed. No one should have to search for information while their loved one is fighting to survive. And now we know that SJS is nowhere near as rare as we were led to believe.

Once we put our website up, they came. Like the movie "Field of Dreams," "If you build it, they will come"—they came from around the world. Some were from five miles from us in Colorado. One was a 6-year-old girl. She got SJS from amoxicillin for an ear infection. Luckily, she was given only two doses of the antibiotic before emergency room doctors realized that she was having a re-action to it and stopped giving it. So, thankfully, her long-term side effects were minimal. Another little girl, less fortunate, from five miles away in the exact opposite direction, got SJS from an over-the-counter ibuprofen product. She was 12 years old when it happened. Now she is 27. She was so disabled from SJS that she ended up having a stroke. She's paralyzed on one side; she's still on a feeding tube to this day; and she is completely blind.

These are medications that we think we can take. We think they're safe. But even reading the package insert will not necessarily warn people strongly enough about SJS, because many of these in-serts just warn of a possible "rash." In some cases, a "rash" is an ap-propriate description of the side effects a person experiences. But it does not describe the horror of SJS. In the cases of package inserts for prescription drugs, like anti-seizure medications, the inserts will say that "in rare instances," SJS may occur. As we have found out the hard way, SJS is not quite so rare.

People who contact us obviously have a loved one who has SJS. SJS is not out in the open, and this is wrong. We're consumers, and we have an over-the-counter product like ibuprofen for our chil-dren—children's ibuprofen—that we can walk into a store without even asking a doctor, pick it up, purchase it, take it home, and give it to our kid. If the kid has a fever, we give it to her, thinking it will reduce that fever. With SJS, one of the first problems is that the fever starts to go up. So parents reach for that product again. Now they've given it to them again. Now, we've basically poured gasoline on a fire.

There is no stopping it. The problem is that SJS is not widely recognized because physicians are taught that it's rare. And believe me, I hear from people from all across the US and all around the world, every single day, sometimes in the middle of the night. SJS is not rare. What is rare is having it reported to the FDA. We need to make sure that these cases are reported so that doctors and our government will start to take it seriously.

Our group is getting better known all the time. Julie appeared on the Montel Williams Show in 2006. (http://www.sjsupport.org/press_releases/Oct_25_2006.html) She was selected by the Denver National Federation of the Blind to meet with Michelle Obama at the Governor's mansion in November 2009 as part of a mentoring program. (http://www.adams50.org/1947101112134057820/blank/browse.asp?a=383&BMDRN=2000&BCOB=0&c=56406) Of course, she handed Mrs. Obama a fact sheet about SJS. Recently, Julie's story was featured on the Discovery Health Channel's "Mystery Diagnosis." (http://www.seopressreleases.com/babys-fight-life-teens-story-survival/7216) And in 2010, she received the Metropolitan Mayors and Commissioners Youth Award. (http://www.ci.westminster.co.us/agendas/ag030810.pdf) The program recognizes youth who have "overcome personal adversity and made positive changes in their lives." I am so proud of her. I think she has my spirit. But I think that spirit is so much more amazing in a young person, especially one who has been through as much as she has.

I am so happy to have this opportunity to tell people about the Ketogenic Diet. I know that it saved Julie's life. In a majority of the calls we get at the SJS Foundation that are about children, the culprits are anti-seizure medications. The worst offender is lamotrigine, which even has a Black Box warning, saying that it can cause SJS. But doctors still prescribe it for children. (Editor's note: For a definition of "black box warning," see http://drugs.about.com/od/bdrugandmedicalterms/g/blackboxdef.htm.)

Whenever a parent calls me about a child whose SJS was caused by an anti-seizure medication, I tell them about the Ketogenic Diet, this wonderful, non-toxic alternative to drugs. I can't tell you how grateful these parents are for this information. They should have learned about the diet from their doctors as soon as their child had his or her first seizure. But they didn't. They only learn about it from me, after their child has experienced one of the worst "side effects" imaginable: SJS. And SJS is a "side effect" that can ruin (or end) their children's lives.

Since we started the foundation and Julie's story has gotten out, SJS has gotten quite a bit of publicity. But unfortunately, most of that publicity neglects to even mention the diet, even though we always tell the interviewer that it was the Ketogenic Diet that saved Julie's life. Most recently, when our story was told on "Mystery Diagnosis," the diet wasn't mentioned, even though I told the producers about it in great detail. That part of our story landed on the cutting room floor. So, I hope that, through Julia Schopick's book, more parents will learn about it.

You may learn more about Jean's organization, The Stevens Johnson Syndrome Foundation at http://www.sjsupport.org/.

In the next section, you will learn about another treatment, Low Dose Naltrexone (LDN). As with the Ketogenic Diet, this treatment has saved many lives, and is, unfortunately, also discovered too late—after the patient has already suffered side effects from the prescribed medications, and from the effects of the disease.

Chapter 11 was contributed by David Gluck, MD, Dr. Bihari's colleague. And in Chapters 12-14, you'll hear from two patients and one family member who finally found LDN. I hope you'll be fascinated by their stories.

Low Dose Naltrexone (LDN)

Low Dose Naltrexone (LDN)

I believe that Low Dose Naltrexone (LDN) is, without a doubt, one of the most important medical discoveries of the twentieth century—if not *the* most important. It certainly is the cheapest and most versatile of the treatments profiled in this book. And that it works for so many conditions is nothing short of remarkable.

LDN is an inexpensive nightly pill, whose main side effect is "vivid dreams." Since naltrexone has been "off-patent" for many years, no company controls it, it is inexpensive to create, and any compounding pharmacist can create it. However, there are several pharmacists that are known to compound it correctly; they are listed on Dr. David Gluck's LDN website at http://www. lowdosenaltrexone.org/comp_pharm.htm and also at http://LDNaware. org/. And more names are being added all the time. (For an excellent article about why choosing the right compounding pharmacy is critical, read http://www.suite101.com/content/where-to-buy-low-dose-naltrexone---ldn-a206700.)

A narcotic blocker, naltrexone was approved by the FDA in the mid-1980s for treating drug and alcohol addiction. Soon afterward, neurologist Bernard Bihari, MD discovered that, in small doses (one-tenth to one-twentieth the dose prescribed for addicts), Low Dose Naltrexone has immune-system-modulating and endorphin-raising capabilities. He reasoned that because of this, it could help patients with immunologically related disorders. He was right. When patients took LDN at bedtime, Dr. Bihari found that it raised their endorphin levels, resulting in halting further progression of their diseases.

Dr. Bihari first began prescribing LDN to his patients with HIV/AIDS. For a great many of them, it stopped their disease from progressing. He reasoned that, since HIV/AIDS was a disease that resulted from a compromised immune system, it would probably work on autoimmune diseases, as well. So he began prescribing LDN for people with multiple sclerosis, lupus and rheumatoid arthritis. Many of these patients, too, experienced no further disease progression. Dr. Bihari also had considerable success using LDN with patients with some cancers that had failed to respond to standard treatments.

In some cases, the results have been truly amazing. For instance, some MS patients, like Vicki Finlayson, have gone from being nearly bedbound, to returning to a totally normal life. In 2008, three years after starting LDN, Vicki was able to walk fifty-three miles to the California State Capitol from her home in Auburn, California to publicize her recovery. (http://www.suite101. com/content/focus-on-low-dose-naltrexone-a54293) At around the same time, she was also able to get off disability and return to work. For other patients, like Noel Bradley, Linda Elsegood and Malcolm West, although their changes haven't been as dramatic, they have nonetheless been significant. Linda and Malcolm write about their experiences in Chapters 12 and 14. And Noel's wife, Mary, writes about their experiences in Chapter 13.

Since the 1980s, several thousand patients have taken LDN for other diseases, too, including Crohn's disease, chronic fatigue syndrome and fibromyalgia. As you learned in Section 2, Dr. Burt Berkson now uses LDN, in combination with intravenous alpha lipoic acid, to bring about remissions in some very serious cancers, including pancreatic cancer, which is considered one of the deadliest forms of the disease. (See Paul Marez's story, Chapter 6.)

Like the other treatments included in this book, patients usually find out about LDN on the Internet, after they have already been prescribed—and been disappointed by—the more toxic drugs. Finding LDN online isn't as difficult as it once was; there are now several websites, and just as many online forums and chat groups, totally devoted to discussions about LDN. (See the Appendix for a sampling.) But this was not the case when Linda Elsegood and Mary Boyle Bradley found LDN years ago.

Many medical doctors have personally observed positive results in their patients who are taking LDN, and some are now even conducting their own small trials of LDN. But the majority of doctors still opt to prescribe the more toxic, side-effect-laden drugs—many of which don't work at all well for their patients. And many still refuse to prescribe LDN.

Surveys and Studies

Many patient surveys have been conducted, and continue to be conducted, on LDN. Three statistically valid user surveys consistently point to 80-85 percent efficacy of LDN in preventing exacerbations of their disease. My e-book, *The Faces of Low Dose Naltrexone*, contains information about these surveys on pages 54-66. (http://www.honestmedicine.com/2009/09/free-ebook-now-available-for-international-ldn-awareness-week-the-faces-of-low-dose-naltrexone.html)

Surveys, studies and patient experience all point to the fact that LDN appears to be most effective when taken early in a disease's progression. Yet few neurologists will prescribe it then. In fact, hardly any will even mention it to a newly diagnosed MS patient. Unfortunately, as I mentioned before, most neurologists are more likely to prescribe the side-effect-laden pharmaceuticals. They most often turn first to the C.R.A.B. drugs, then to the very dangerous Tysabri. (Editor's note: The C.R.A.B. drugs are so named because of their acronym: Copaxone, Rebif, Avonex and Betaseron.) Some doctors, as you will learn from Malcolm West's chapter, even have their patients undergo chemotherapy or massive blood transfusions (plasmapherisis), before prescribing LDN.

Two successful studies on LDN treatment for multiple sclerosis were presented at the Annual Meeting of the American Academy of Neurology in April 2007:

- One from the University of California at San Francisco (UCSF): http://painsandiego.files.wordpress.com/2009/05/ldn-in-ms-bruce-cree-md_-2008-ucsf-poster.pdf
- And one from Milan: http://www.ncbi.nlm.nih.gov/pubmed/1872 8058?ordinalpos=5&itool=EntrezSystem2.PEntrez.Pubmed.Pubmed_ ResultsPanel.Pubmed_DefaultReportPanel.Pubmed_RVDo

For a more complete listing of LDN trials, please go to Dr. David Gluck's and SammyJo Wilkinson's websites:

- Dr. Gluck's site: http://www.lowdosenaltrexone.org
- SammyJo's site: http://www.LDNers.org

Resources

Several books have been written about LDN, including *Up the Creek With a Paddle* by Mary Bradley; *The Promise of Low Dose Naltrexone* by SammyJo Wilkinson and Elaine Moore; and *Google LDN* by Joseph Wouk, author Herman Wouk's son.

So far there have been five LDN conferences in the United States and two in Scotland. In October 2010, another conference was held in England.

During the first International Low Dose Naltrexone Awareness Week (ILDNAW), in October 2009, LDN patient advocates from around the world worked together to spread the word about this inexpensive, off-label use of the generic drug they credit with their improvement. And Linda Elsegood (LDN Research Trust) hired an excellent public relations firm, which spread the word about LDN throughout the UK and beyond. Most of these media placements are listed (with hyperlinks) in Chapter 12.

Cost

As I have mentioned several times throughout this book, it troubles me greatly that people find it so difficult to get effective, low-cost treatments like the ones I am profiling. But, almost as troubling to me is the fact that our insurance companies are paying out exorbitant amounts of money for pharmaceutical treatments for autoimmune disorders—medications that are often much less effective than LDN, and have many more side effects. Yet, they will not pay for LDN. (Editor's note: As you will learn in Linda Elsegood's chapter, in the UK, the cost of LDN for some patients is covered by the National Health Service.)

Let's compare the cost of the drugs doctors most often prescribe for MS patients—the C.R.A.B. drugs and Tysabri—with the cost of LDN.

On the one hand, Low Dose Naltrexone costs anywhere from $25 to $40 per month, depending on the dose you are taking, and the compounding pharmacy you buy the LDN from. By comparison, typically, MS drugs cost $1,000-$2,000 per month, sometimes more, an increase by at least forty to fifty times the cost of LDN.

In her July 21, 2009 posting on the About.com MS site, Julie Stachowiak, PhD, looks at the rise in cost for the five main MS drugs in a two-year period, from 2007 to 2009: http://ms.about. com/b/2009/07/21/multiple-sclerosis-drug-prices-whoa.htm. Not only are these drugs expensive, but, as you can see, their prices have increased rapidly.

- Avonex (was $10,000/year): Minimum price = $23,736; Maximum price = $30,660

- Betaseron (was $10,000/year): Minimum price = $22,272; Maximum price = $32,616

- Copaxone (was $10,000/year): Minimum price = $23,208; Maximum price = $33,804

- Rebif (was $15,600/year): Minimum price = $25,068; Maximum price = $30,756

- Tysabri (was $28,400/year), now costs $31,332 for the drug itself, with additional charges for the infusion facility or clinic fees.

To give you an example of the savings that can be realized by taking LDN instead of one of the C.R.A.B. drugs, let's suppose an MS patient pays for LDN at the high end of the scale at $40/month. That's $480/year. The minimum annual price of Avonex ($23,736) is nearly fifty times the price of LDN. The maximum annual price of Avonex ($30,660) is approximately 62.5 times the annual price of LDN.

These shocking figures are similar for all the other most-often-prescribed MS drugs.

Considering that naltrexone was proven to be safe at 50 mg twenty-six years ago by the FDA, and that people take Low Dose Naltrexone at 4.5 mg (sometimes even lower), doesn't it make sense to try LDN first—before trying these other drugs?

It seems to make sense to lots of happy patients, and to an ever-growing number of practicing doctors!

The Experts

While this is the only section of the book that doesn't include the personal story of the treatment in the words of that treatment's pioneer, you will hear from David Gluck, MD (Chapter 11), Dr.

Bihari's childhood friend and colleague. As you will see, it is Dr. Bihari's story, too, since Dr. Gluck literally lived through it with Dr. Bihari. I think you will find his take on LDN fascinating.

Unfortunately, Dr. Bihari, whom I and many others consider to be the LDN hero and pioneer, died on May 16, 2010, while this book was being written. (See HonestMedicine.com's memorial tribute to him at http://www.honestmedicine.com/2010/05/bernard-bihari-md-november-11-1931-to-may-16-20100518.html.) Thanks to his perseverance for over twenty-five years and his success with treating patients throughout those years, there are now several physicians around the world who are using LDN to treat autoimmune (and other) diseases.

In the Appendix, I am including links to videos and audios featuring some of the doctors who prescribe and advocate for LDN, as well as links to some of their websites. They are prescribing this low-cost, very effective medication for their patients because it is helping them. LDN certainly isn't making any of these doctors a great deal of money.

LDN Advocates/Chapter Contributors

I found it nearly impossible to choose which of the many LDN patient advocates' stories I would include in this book. I finally settled on Linda Elsegood, Mary Boyle Bradley and Malcolm West because, in addition to having their own fascinating personal stories to tell, each of them is actively involved in promoting the use of LDN through their own organizations, websites and books—and in one case, even through an Internet radio program, devoted one hundred percent to LDN. They are all devoting a significant (always unpaid) portion of their lives to getting the word out to more people with MS, so that other patients won't have to go through the pain and misery they went through before finding LDN.

- Chapter 12: LDN patient Linda Elsegood, whose UK charity organization, www.LDNResearchTrust.org, has been extremely successful in getting the word out about LDN in the UK. There are several other UK organizations, as well. There is no way I could ever list all of them; there are far too many, both in the UK and the US.

- Chapter 13: Mary Boyle Bradley has written *Up the Creek With a Paddle*, and also has had an Internet radio show, devoted to getting the word out about LDN. Her show aired on a weekly basis from April 28, 2009 to January 10, 2010. During that time, it had several thousand downloads per week. In total, it has been downloaded approximately 33,000 times. Mary's show no longer airs on a regular basis, but she plans to conduct more interviews "as big LDN events unfold." You may listen to her past shows by going to this website: http://www.blogtalkradio.com/mary-boyle-bradley.

- Chapter 14: For years, Malcolm West was treated with three of the C.R.A.B. drugs (Avonex, Rebif and Copaxone), as well as with Tysabri and chemotherapy. None of these medications worked. It was only when he lost his job—and with it, his health insurance—that Malcolm finally tried LDN. His condition began to improve almost immediately. Along with Sherri Shelton White, another LDN patient advocate, Malcolm is one of the driving forces behind LDN Aware: http://LDNaware.org/. When it is completed, LDN Aware promises to be the umbrella website, uniting all the LDN resources from around the world. This is a huge undertaking. Malcolm was the linchpin who got it started.

Now on to the personal stories.

CHAPTER 11

David Gluck, MD

An LDN Champion (Dr. Bihari's Colleague)

Dr. David Gluck is a childhood friend of Dr. Bernard Bihari, the neurologist who pioneered the use of LDN for autoimmune diseases. One of today's best-known champions of LDN, Dr. Gluck has been a board-certified specialist in both internal and preventive medicine for many years, and believes that LDN is one of the most significant therapeutic discoveries in fifty years. He and his son, Joel, manage the not-for-profit website: www. LDNinfo.org. By freely distributing LDN information via their website, the Glucks have helped thousands of people get their lives back. I am delighted that Dr. Gluck has agreed to write this chapter.

I first heard about LDN from my good friend, Bernard Bihari, the neurologist who pioneered the use of LDN in clinical practice. Dr. Bihari and I were kids together and grew up together. He went to Harvard Medical College; I went to Cornell Medical College. In the mid-1980s, Dr. Bihari was running the Alcohol and Drug Abuse section at Downstate Medical Center in Brooklyn where he began to experiment with a very low dose of the drug, naltrexone. Naltrexone had been approved by the FDA in 1984 for treating people with addiction problems. Dr. Bihari was experimenting with treating people with LDN who had a disease that was unnamed at the time. That disease turned out to be HIV/AIDS.

He had great success with it in a small clinical trial. But he had difficulty publishing his work. However, on the strength of what he found, he went into private practice to try to bring this treatment to the people who were suffering from this new disease. A few years later, he started treating patients with autoimmune diseases, also with great success.

I have come to think that LDN is one of the most significant therapeutic discoveries in fifty years. LDN is absolutely unique. And that's part of its problem, in that it's a brand new paradigm, a new way of thinking of treatment. Instead of the medication actually doing the work, LDN goes into the body and essentially tricks the body by forcing it to double and triple its output of endorphins and metenkephalin, also known as opioid growth factor (OGF). (http://en.wikipedia.org/wiki/Met-enkephalin) Those endorphins and metenkephalin, in turn, cause the immune system to strengthen. A nice way to think about LDN is that it is not like any other medication whatsoever. It is a way to strengthen the immune system.

The reason why this is so vital is because studies have shown that autoimmune diseases are all marked by a weak, dysfunctional immune system. The moment the immune system is strengthened by LDN, it remembers that its first and most important job is to never attack itself. When you are stuck with a weak immune system, a dysfunctional immune system, you often get these autoimmune diseases. By taking LDN, the diseases stop progressing because the immune system now is strengthened, so it no longer attacks "self." No further symptoms, no further attacks. And that happens with the vast majority of people using LDN. Naturally, HIV/AIDS is a problem that has a dysfunctional immune system. Here again, LDN helps. It also helps many cancers.

Dr. Burton Berkson has done some very impressive work treating several cancers, including the most recalcitrant—Stage IV pancreatic cancer—with a combination of LDN and intravenous alpha lipoic acid. For more information, see "The Long-Term Survival of a Patient With Pancreatic Cancer With Metastases to the Liver After Treatment With the Intravenous α-Lipoic Acid/Low-Dose Naltrexone Protocol." Berkson BM, Rubin DM, Berkson AJ. *Integr. Cancer Ther.* Vol. 5, No. 1, 83-89 (2006) (http://ict.sagepub.com/cgi/content/short/5/1/83) and "Revisiting the ALA/N [alpha-lipoic acid/low-dose naltrexone] protocol for people with metastatic and non-metastatic pancreatic cancer: a report of 3 new cases." Berkson BM, Rubin DM, Berkson AJ. *Integr. Cancer Ther.* 2009 Dec;8(4):416-22.) (http://ict.sagepub.com/cgi/content/abstract/8/4/416)

LDN helps a broad spectrum of diseases, not only autoimmune diseases, but any illness based on a disturbed and weak immune system, which essentially is the description of every autoimmune disease out there. There are probably a couple of hundred autoimmune diseases. Of course, LDN doesn't work all the time. There are bound to be exceptions. Nothing works one hundred percent of the time. But it's better than anything we've ever had going. It's a very, very impressive therapy.

Even diseases that aren't generally recognized in medicine as being clearly autoimmune are showing significant benefits from taking LDN—for example, the motor neuron diseases, like primary lateral sclerosis or amyotrophic lateral sclerosis (ALS, also known as Lou Gehrig's disease). We've had a significant number of reports from people in Australia who have formed a group to help each other with these illnesses. The only reports they've ever seen of people with ALS saying, "Wow, that's been helpful to me," are those who have tried LDN. In addition, people with Parkinson's disease tend not to progress further once they start taking LDN. (For ALS and Parkinson's references see http://www.lowdosenaltrexone.org/others.htm and search for "Gehrig" and "Parkinson's.")

People worry about the possible short-term and long-term side effects of taking LDN because there have been so many past stories of other so-called treatments that have had bad side effects. Again,

LDN is remarkable. What you're taking when you take naltrexone is a pure narcotic blocker. That's all that it does. With LDN, you're taking a tiny dose, so that each day it's only in your system for perhaps four or five hours. The rest of the day it's not there. Let's say you take it at bedtime. (You don't have to take it then, but it's proven to be a good way to use it.) You're blocking the opioid receptors, the narcotic receptors in your body, which are also the endorphin receptors. When you block them for a few hours, by the time you wake up in the morning, the blockade is gone, and your body has doubled and tripled its endorphin production.

Many people know about the endorphins. For instance, vigorous running will turn on endorphins; others claim that even dark chocolate turns them on. But in my experience, nothing does it as successfully as LDN. I say this because I've been using it for over seven years now. So has every adult member of my family and many, many of my friends. They all report that the common cold has become virtually a thing of the past. If they wake up in the morning with some minor symptoms of a cold, the symptoms tend to be gone by the afternoon. I think that medicine has been waiting for a way to safely strengthen the immune system for all these years, and I think we've finally got it.

People ask if there is an initial period of time where patients have to adjust to LDN. I tell them that once LDN gets the respect from medicine that it deserves, and gets the studies that it requires, we'll find out the answers to many questions people have about it. But there's no correct answer right now. Most people start out without taking lower doses; they just jump into the 4.5 mg dose, and they're fine. The occasional exception would be the person with multiple sclerosis (MS) who already has had quite a problem with muscular spasms, and it is recommended that those people use only 3 mg.

I'm often asked, if LDN is so wonderful, why doctors are so leery about prescribing it. I tell them that it requires a good deal of empathy to understand why that's so. You have to put yourself in the position of the physician. The physician has spent years and years in training. And that training focuses on the scientific method, on making sure that what he is going to use has been shown to work in a scientific way backed up by scientific studies—not from patient stories, which they call "anecdotes." To them, it's got to be in a well-known medical journal; it's got to be peer-reviewed. To them, it has to be tested in large studies—double-blind, placebo-controlled studies. It has to be FDA-approved. But even if it's not FDA-approved for a particular use, doctors do have the right to write an off-label prescription for any dose of something that has been FDA-approved, even if it was approved at a higher dose, like naltrexone was.

Naltrexone was approved by the FDA for heroin addicts in the early 1980s, and in later years, was further approved for use with alcoholics. So, even though every doctor has a perfect right to write the prescription for LDN, he still hasn't really seen it in his medical journals as a treatment for autoimmune diseases.

And why is that? He hasn't seen it in the medical journals because to run the big studies costs millions of dollars. To get something approved at the level that the FDA needs to see it can cost tens or hundreds of millions of dollars. Some people estimate it costs a half a billion dollars. The large pharmaceutical firms are essentially the only ones who have that sort of money. The government used to do more of the medical research, but its funding was cut in the 1980s. Now big drug studies are mostly done by the pharmaceutical companies. (Editor's note: For more information on this topic, see "Dr. John Abramson's *Overdosed America: The Broken Promise of American Medicine*—OR, How Medical Research Lost Its Credibility" on HonestMedicine.com: http://www.honestmedicine.com/2008/10/abramson.html.)

Naltrexone has been off-patent for some years. Pharmaceutical companies run in the other direction when people talk about wanting to run a trial for LDN, because they would put in all that money and find that there are no profits waiting at the other end, since anybody can get the generic naltrexone and break it down into whatever dose they want through a compounding pharmacy at a very low cost.

Still, there have been some very impressive LDN trials. A lot of them have been done through individuals who have been helped by LDN, and who have made gifts to their local medical centers. They're very small trials, though, and aren't the big trials that are generally looked for by physicians. If you'll check my website, www.LDNinfo.org, we list all the details about the clinical studies and the clinical trials that have been accomplished.

In 2007, there was a trial run on LDN for MS by Dr. Bruce Cree at the University of California, San Francisco. The results were reported as a board presentation at the international MS meetings in Montreal in the summer of 2008. The clinical trial was double-blind. Though it was a good clinical trial, it was brief, given that all they had was $25,000 in the way of contributions. Vicki Finlayson, a wonderful LDN advocate whose MS was virtually cured by LDN, organized the event to raise that money.

Finally, in 2010, I am delighted to report that the University of California, San Francisco's Neurology Department has published the information in the February 19, 2010 *Annals of Neurology*, "Pilot trial of Low Dose Naltrexone and quality of life in MS." (http://www.ptsr.org.pl/pl/files/20100223_1312/001_LDN_paper_Annals_of_Neurology_110.pdf)

Hopefully, now many thousands of people suffering from MS will be able to turn to that publication and bring it to their own specialist and say, "Please, write me a prescription for this."

There have been other LDN studies, including one at Penn State with Crohn's disease: http://www.ncbi.nlm.nih.gov/pubmed/17222 320?itool=EntrezSystem2.PEntrez.Pubmed.Pubmed_ResultsPanel.Pubmed_RVDocSum&ordinalpos=1. Again, the results were very positive, as they were in many other studies, including one in Italy and another in Mali, Africa. In fact, none of the studies conducted on LDN have found it wanting.

A big part of the problem for getting approval for new drugs is the way that the system was set up in the United States. When this system was first set up, nobody anticipated that there would ever be such a thing as LDN, a much-needed but already out-of-patent drug, which offered no possible profits for a pharmaceutical company. If somebody comes up with an amazing therapeutic discovery and it happens to be a discovery that offers no profits to pharmaceutical companies, it just can't find its way to the FDA for approval. Therefore, it also will not be published in an important medical journal, because for that to happen, a drug must first go through rigorous, very expensive trials that only pharmaceutical companies or the government can afford. A vicious cycle. (Editor's note: More about FDA and its approval process can be found at http://en.wikipedia.org/wiki/Food_and_Drug_Administration.)

My sense is that we've stuck ourselves, unexpectedly, in a system where the pharmaceutical companies have become the gatekeepers, so to speak, as to what the public gets to hear about, and what they get to have as a new therapy. The pharmaceutical companies simply put aside anything that has no profit potential.

Right now, thinking of MS, it's just terrible to think about the standard drugs, which tend to be injectables, because they all have awful side effects and don't have much to offer in the way of help. And they are all terribly, terribly expensive. In contrast, this little capsule, LDN, taken by mouth once a night, costs less than a dollar a day. And it has no significant side effects.

People with autoimmune diseases often look for specialists to write a prescription for LDN. But because specialists are suspicious of any medication that has not appeared in their own journals, I usually tell them that they would do better going to their general practitioner (GP) or family physician. When the GP or family doctor looks up naltrexone in the *Physicians' Desk Reference*®, he'll say, "Well, let's see ... naltrexone 50 mg. Well, there are no significant side effects. What do you want, 4.5 mg? Well, that can't hurt you." And he'll write them the prescription. People can save lots of time by going to their GP or family doctor.

When people write to our website, we refer them to the nearly 8,000 members of the LDN Yahoo Group, who have been wonderfully helpful. (For more information, see: http://health.groups.yahoo. com/group/lowdosenaltrexone.) Many of them keep lists of physicians who they know are happy to write LDN prescriptions. I know that Skip's Pharmacy in Boca Raton has made a commitment to sharing the names of doctors in Florida who have helped people with LDN prescriptions.

When people write to our website, we send them the addresses of those physician groups whose members are especially interested in treating people with complementary and alternative treatments. I don't really think, though, that LDN is a complementary or alternative treatment because it's just a very low dose of an FDA-approved medication.

There is only one thing people need to be concerned about with LDN. They must know that they cannot begin even this tiny dose of naltrexone if they regularly take a narcotic-containing pain medication. If you are dependent on a narcotic medication, and then take LDN, you will likely go into a very, very difficult withdrawal reaction. So, to that extent, of course, you have to be weaned off by your doctor over a ten-day to two-week period before you can think about starting LDN. Other than that, the few cautions, the very few cautions, are listed on the website: http://www.lowdosenaltrexone.org.

I am such a strong believer in the power of LDN that I sincerely believe that its widespread use could change healthcare. When I first learned that President Obama had set aside a substantial amount of money to fund Comparative Effectiveness Research trials to compare the efficacy of existing drugs with new ones, I immediately thought of LDN. (http://www.hhs.gov/recovery/programs/cer/) If such a trial were done, comparing LDN to some of the more expensive MS drugs, I have no doubt that LDN would come out the clear winner.

For over a year now (as of February 2010), I have been working hard to reach people in Washington, DC, who are involved in trying to change our healthcare system. I assumed those government people, from the President on down to key administrators for health care reform to related members of Congress, would be interested in learning about LDN because they have often stated publicly that they want to improve the system, so that more people will have access to good care. They have also said that we need to reduce costs. With both of these goals in mind, I would think that they would be especially interested in learning about a treatment like LDN, which is both effective and inexpensive.

One of my friends, an intellectual property attorney, has taken LDN to heart. Through his firm, he's helped me make contact with a group of people close to one of the congresswomen in Washington from our area (the New York City metropolitan area). One of her aides spoke with the attorney and me and asked us to send him lots of information about LDN. We did, including information about LDN's safety, and concrete statistics on how LDN could save the system a huge amount of money. (http://ms.about.com/b/2009/07/21/multiple-sclerosis-drug-prices-whoa.htm) The aide assured us that while healthcare isn't really this congressperson's area, she would send our information to others who are involved. I've also personally written to every person in the White House staff involved in the healthcare fight.

My point, of course, is that LDN is a wonderful way to reduce costs, while increasing health. I'm confused, though, because I thought that was what our new administration in Washington was going to try to do. I was very hopeful that they would be anxious to learn about LDN. But now, since I've heard nothing, I'd have to say that I'm somewhat discouraged. Nevertheless, I intend to keep trying.

~

This chapter was adapted from an interview Dr. Gluck gave to Mary Bradley on her BlogTalkRadio program. To hear the interview, please go to http://www.blogtalkradio.com/mary-boyle-bradley/2009/05/05/dr-david-gluck-live-on-the-mary-bradley-show-talking-about-low-dose-naltrexone-ldn.

I spoke recently with Dr. Gluck, and he told me that, although he is discouraged, he is not ready to give up. He reiterated his hope that someone who is reading this book may know how to get in the front door of a Senator or a member of the House of Representatives. He has lots of information to share with them about LDN. If you would like to help Dr. Gluck in his mission to get LDN considered for Comparative Effectiveness Research trials, please contact him for more information at email@lowdosenaltrexone.org.

In the next three chapters, you will learn about three patients' successful efforts to get LDN and the positive results they achieved with it.

CHAPTER 12

Linda Elsegood, UK

LDN Advocate: A Tribute to Persistence

I first spoke with Linda Elsegood (via Skype) when a group of us were planning the publicity for the first International Low Dose Naltrexone Awareness Week in October 2009. Very soon, I knew she and I would be friends for life. Her sense of humor, her unstoppable nature and her amazing spirit all combined to make her someone to admire. In the weeks and months that followed, I watched Linda in total amazement as she single-handedly got the media in the UK and beyond to take notice of LDN. She has gotten more media placements than any one person involved in the LDN movement. The fact that Linda has MS and can accomplish so much is a tribute to Linda, and to LDN.

The following is her first-hand account of her journey, adapted and expanded with permission, from an interview with Mary Bradley on her Internet radio show.

(http://www.blogtalkradio.com/mary-boyle-bradley)

By the time I was diagnosed with MS in August 2000, I was very, very sick. I had had MS for at least twelve years, without the doctors knowing it. I'd been having numbness, pins and needles, things that came and went. And I'd go to my doctors and say, "Look, for some reason or another, my calf muscle in my right leg goes numb and I can't feel it." And he said, "Ahhh, it's no

problem. You've got a slipped disc." Then I had electric shocks going down to my fingertips when I put my chin down. The doctor
said that was a trapped nerve in my neck. But, in hindsight, these
were all MS symptoms. Once I got the diagnosis, I could actually
go back and see that I had had MS for a long time.

I was initially given a course of intravenous steroids, which did
absolutely nothing for me. Six weeks later, the neurologist was very
concerned. I had optic neuritis on top of all the other symptoms,
and my double vision was really bad. I had no hearing whatsoever
in my left ear; that ear was totally dead. The neurologist said that
he was worried that I was going to become blind and deaf, and he
wanted to do another course of intravenous steroids. The prospect
of being deaf and blind was very scary. So I didn't object, and took
the intravenous steroids. In a few weeks, they started to work very
slightly, but I wasn't anywhere near back to normal. Later on, I was
offered Rebif, which I took for eight months. That is the whole
story as to what I was offered drug-wise.

After the second course of steroids, I asked my doctor, "How
long do you think it will be before I'll start feeling better?"

He said to me, "Well, to be honest, I think if you were going to
feel better, you would have done so by now."

I wasn't really living. I was just surviving. There was nothing else
that I was being offered.

I was desperate to find something that was going to help me. I
saw my neurologist in October 2003. He told me I was secondary
progressive MS and there was nothing more that could be done for
me. I had tried everything. What else could I do? So I sat at the
computer and started to research online. But with a patch over one
eye, I could only be online for a few minutes at a time.

Then I found LDN. It took me several weeks to really research
it and find some people who were taking it. The conclusion I came
to was that if it wasn't going to do me any good, it certainly wasn't

going to do me any harm. Everyone said, "What have you got to lose by trying it?" That was what I decided I was going to do. I contacted Dr. Bob Lawrence, who gave me a fact sheet that I printed off and took to my own general practitioner, who was very interested. She said that she was unable to prescribe it for me, but that if I got it privately, she would be happy to monitor me. That's what happened. I managed to get LDN and she monitored me.

I didn't have any side effects at all. Now, I was actually disappointed about that. I mean, people don't like side effects in drugs, but I wanted side effects. I'd been told that I'd probably get vivid dreams. I might have constipation. I might have worsening of pre-existing symptoms. I just wanted to know it was working. I wanted something to happen. I could have been taking paracetamol (acetaminophen or Tylenol in the US). It did nothing. I thought to myself that this was my last chance of trying to become me again, and it wasn't going to work. Then, hey, presto! It was such a big surprise when three weeks later, things started to improve.

First, I improved cognitively. The feeling of this fogging in my head had been very difficult at the time. I couldn't see properly. I couldn't hear properly. It was scary, the way I was deteriorating to the point where I slurred my speech as though I'd had a stroke. I had to chew my food carefully. But I'd still start to choke on it. People had to pound me on the back. I couldn't think properly. It was as though English had become my second language. I would be trying to think of a word and it would make sense to me. I knew what I wanted to say, but what actually came out of my mouth was something totally different. It was as if I was suffering from Alzheimer's or something. I just couldn't say what I wanted to say. That was the most scary, frightening thing ever. But suddenly, after taking LDN for three weeks, everything became clear. I could think again. I started to hear, started to see, started to feel like "me" again.

While this fogging in my head cleared in three weeks, the other symptoms took longer to disappear, mainly the restless legs. You know, the burning limbs where you feel that you're on fire, as though you've been out in the sun. You're sunburned and you can't cool your limbs down. But when I actually touched my legs, they felt cold. They weren't burning. But inside, they felt as if they were on fire. Finally that went away, and the numbness and the pins and needles went, and the twitching muscles went. In bed at night, my legs used to slash around all over the place; they just wouldn't lie still. Of course, since I hadn't been able to sleep properly, I'd felt fatigued all the time. After taking LDN, as time went on, my legs started slowly to move less and less in bed, and I got more rest.

I must say, if I hadn't found LDN when I did, I don't think I'd be here today.

I've been taking LDN for nearly five-and-a-half years. My quality of life is very good, but I'm still not pre-MS Linda. I still know I've got MS. I'm still limited in doing certain things. But with the quality of life I have now, I can set goals. I can achieve them. I can feel I'm contributing. I'm not just surviving. I'm not just trying to get from waking up in the morning until bedtime, which was what my life was like before. I couldn't set any goals. I couldn't even wash myself. I couldn't brush my hair. I couldn't walk, couldn't think, couldn't talk—you name it.

Even though I was feeling so much better, my neurologist didn't believe that my improvement was due to LDN. I was ecstatic, though. I was saying, "Isn't it great? Isn't this LDN wonderful?"

My neurologist said, "No, it's not the LDN. When we said you were secondary progressive MS, we made a mistake. You're still 'relapsing remitting,' and you're in remission now." Even though he didn't think it was the LDN that was working, he said I should continue to take it. "Well, whatever you're doing, don't stop it," my neurologist added.

I suppose that's the nearest you are going to get to a neurologist admitting that it is the LDN. But they're still not prescribing it for other MS patients, which is a shame.

My MS journey had been so difficult, so tiring. It had taken me such a long time to find the LDN. So, when I was feeling able, I wanted to sing the praises of LDN from the rooftops. I wanted to let people know about LDN who were in the same position that I was in, and yet who might even be worse than I was, who weren't able to fight the MS because they were so ill. I wanted to fight for them. I wanted to say, "Hey, there is something out there. If your doctor or neurologist hasn't told you about it, it doesn't mean to say that it's not out there." I'm always very careful of not saying it's a miracle drug, or that it's a cure, because there are some people, unfortunately, for whom LDN doesn't work. But, what have you got to lose by trying it?

I formed the LDN Research Trust in 2004, and secured registered charity status in the United Kingdom, in order to raise funds to get LDN into clinical trials. We have a website: www.LDNResearchTrust.org. Getting funding has proven to be very difficult: I've written hundreds of letters, made hundreds of phone calls, and gone to many meetings. So far, we have raised £27,000 (the equivalent of about $40,000). But almost from the beginning, people were contacting us, asking how they could obtain LDN.

Instead of just being focused on raising funds for research, we also give patients information about LDN. We tell patients, "If you'd like to try LDN, the first thing is to take this fact sheet to your GP (General Practitioner), who may or may not prescribe it on the NHS (National Health System)." (Editor's note: Examples of information sheets to bring to your doctor are in the Appendix.) If the GP prescribes the LDN on the NHS, then the state pays for it, rather than the patient.

Stephen Dickson, a pharmacist in Scotland, tells us that there are 200 NHS GPs that are prescribing LDN through his pharmacy. I know that there are far more than that who are getting their LDN from other sources. But when I first started, we didn't know of a single neurologist who was in favor of LDN. Now we know of eleven who are not actually prescribing LDN, but who are writing to their patients' GPs, saying that they have no objection to the GPs prescribing LDN for this patient. This is a really big breakthrough.

In my case, I pay for my LDN out of pocket. Other MS patients are getting it paid for them by the NHS, though the majority of people have to buy it themselves.

People often ask me where their money goes if they make a donation to the LDN Research Trust. I tell them that if you specify that you want your money to be used for clinical trials, it will be put aside for clinical trials. The only money that is ever taken out of the charity is for the administrative costs. Nobody ever gets paid. Everybody who is helping works as a volunteer, so every penny that is given to the charity works for the charity. We have to raise money every month. We do have some people who make regular donations, which really helps. But, there are running costs, you know: the website, phone, postage, printing, etc., which have to be funded from somewhere.

We now have our first clinical trial ready to start. It's a trial on the bladder. (Editor's note: Many MS patients have bladder problems.) In April 2009, Dr. Tom Gilhooly was talking about it at the first European LDN conference in Glasgow. He's hoping to get financial support from the CSO's office (Chief Scientist Office) in Scotland, which will be a big help. He would like their backing. Rather than having to find extra funds himself, the CSO's funding would open doors to getting extra funding. We only need £50,000 (British pounds) to get this trial up and running. We're hoping to get the money. As of this writing, it's in phase two of finding out if we've got the funding from them. We have our fingers crossed that we do. Then, thankfully, that trial will be funded.

We're hoping that this small trial will get LDN on the UK map. We would like the National Health Service to do a full trial. It would save the government so much money if they didn't have to pay for patients to take so many of the more expensive MS drugs. If people could actually take LDN, for example, for MS, when they are first diagnosed, and while they still have a high level of fitness, rather than waiting until they have deteriorated, until they're desperate, then they could keep working longer. They wouldn't have to be on benefits. That would be a savings to the government, as well.

Thankfully, LDN is really becoming much better known. In the US, there have been five LDN conferences. Lots of doctors who prescribe LDN to their patients speak at these conferences. So do lots of the patients who have successfully used LDN. The conferences also disseminate information about the trials that have been conducted on LDN, and those trials that are still in the process of being conducted. But until recently, there hadn't been any LDN conferences in Europe. The first one was held in Glasgow in April 2009. It was a great success and was positively buzzing. Its purpose was to reach the media. This was very difficult to do. Only a few newspapers in Scotland ran stories. Dr. Gilhooly was briefly on "This Morning," a daytime television show in the UK, talking about LDN. This UK morning show is similar to the Oprah Show in America; it is the #1 daytime programme in the UK.

But six months later, in October 2009, during the first International LDN Awareness Week (October 19-25), we got a great deal of media attention. (http://www.honestmedicine.com/2009/08/international-ldn-awareness-week-october-1925th-2009.html) The LDN Research Trust hired a public relations firm, and they did a terrific job. There were articles in several publications, including:

- An amazing article in a national paper, *The Daily Express*: http://www.express.co.uk/posts/view/133731/The-drug-that-changed-my-life-should-be-available-to-all. The page uploads on the website were over 2,200 for five days. This was astounding, because page uploads are normally 600 for an entire week!

Other coverage:

- *Let's Talk!*, an East Anglia Magazine that covers six counties in the UK (http://www.ldnresearchtrustfiles.co.uk/docs/1.pdf)

- *The Herald* in Australia (http://www.ldnresearchtrustfiles.co.uk/docs/Article-Hoping%20for%20MS%20cure%20with%20Steely%20Resolve%20The%20Herald%2020%20Oct09.pdf)

- The Isle of Orkney paper (Scotland), *The Orcadian* (http://www.ldnresearchtrustfiles.co.uk/docs/C&C.pdf)

- An article in a Bulgarian publication (http://www.ldnresearchtrustfiles.co.uk/docs/LDNchernomore.jpg)

- Many LDN users were interviewed throughout the UK that week. You may read these articles on the LDN Research Trust's forum under "LDN in the Media and News Updates" at http://forum.ldnresearchtrust.org/index.php?/forum/63-ldn-in-the-media-and-news-updates/page__prune_day__100__sort_by__Z-A__sort_key__last_post__topicfilter__all.

We feel that it's important for the media to take notice of LDN. That's the way patients are going to learn about it. We feel that media coverage is so important that we've actually set up an International LDN Awareness Fund. (http://www.mycharitypage.com/LDN-fund/) At this link, people can donate money to go to PR coverage.

Since the first LDN Awareness Week in October 2009, our work has continued. Media stories have been published, the biggest being in the *British Journal of Neuroscience Nursing*. (http://www.ldnresearchtrustfiles.co.uk/docs/BJNN.pdf) They invited us to submit an article. Dr. Tom Gilhooly, as medical advisor to the Trust, wrote it, and it was accepted for publication. We were so delighted with this piece because it was the first article on LDN to be published in a British medical journal.

Here are a few links to other articles that have been published in the British press after International LDN Awareness Week:

- In the *Leicester Mercury*, "Leicestershire woman in fight for drug to be available on NHS," at http://www.thisisleicestershire. co.uk/news/Leicestershire-woman-fight-drug-available-NHS/article-1552176-detail/article.html

- *The Woking News*, "For me, LDN is life-changing," at http:// www.ldnresearchtrustfiles.co.uk/docs/Woking%20News%20and%20 Mail.pdf

As of April 28, 2010, there are more updates here: http://www. ldnresearchtrustfiles.co.uk/docs/LDN%20Stories.pdf.

In my introduction to this chapter, I wrote that Linda is a whirl-wind of activity on behalf of LDN. I think that her words and media placements prove my point. But one thing that I do not want to go unnoticed is the fact that, because she is "the face" of the LDN Research Trust, Linda spends hours and hours on the phone every day with people who have battled their MS for years, and have just discovered (through her website, or through Facebook) that there is such a drug as LDN out there. Whether these people are angry, depressed, or just seeking information, Linda is there for them. She answers their questions and their concerns, and she helps them to actually get the LDN, by help-ing them find doctors and compounding pharmacists to assist them. Linda has told me that her greatest pleasure is seeing people who had felt hopeless feel hopeful once again, thanks to LDN. (To listen to Mary Boyle Bradley's interview on blog-talkradio, from which this chapter was taken and expanded, please go here: http://www.blogtalkradio.com/mary-boyle-bradley/ 2009/05/19/the-mary-bradley-show. And to purchase a DVD fea-turing presentations from several LDN conferences, go to http:// ldnurl.info/dvd2010.)

CHAPTER 13

Mary Boyle Bradley on LDN

"Thank Goodness for the Internet!"

I have grown close with each and every contributor to this book, and have a very special relationship with each one. Of all of them, I think I relate most personally to Mary, because it was her husband—not Mary herself—who became ill with an incurable disease. And like me with Tim, Mary refused to believe that Noel's situation was hopeless. I still laugh at Mary's assertion that Noel's doctor wrote a prescription for LDN, just to get rid of her. I am sure that Tim's doctors often did the same.

I can also relate to the way Mary took to researching on the Internet ("Thank goodness for the Internet!"), and the way she followed up by phoning people, the way she phoned Dr. Bihari to learn about LDN. In Yiddish, we call that "chutzpah," and I certainly admire it!

Parts of this chapter have been adapted from Mary's book about LDN, *Up the Creek With a Paddle.*

It's my pleasure to introduce Mary; I hope you'll find her as much of an inspiration as I do.

I met Noel in my parents' hotel in Galway, Ireland, when I was twenty-one and he was twenty-five. It was love at first sight. Before we got married, Noel had been feeling numbness in his foot, a numbness that wouldn't go away, and in fact, progressed. At first we joked about it, then we decided to ignore the problem, until we couldn't any longer. Noel's legs had become completely numb from both knees down. He had a staggering gait, and looked like he would fall over with every step. He had to hold onto walls to get around. It was terrifying.

His first neurologist didn't think it was MS. It was my brother Phil, a physician, who was the first to think it probably was MS. I chose not to believe him, and even accused him of having a bad bedside manner! It wasn't until the birth of our first daughter, Annie Kate, that Noel was officially diagnosed with primary progressive MS (PPMS). His neurologist told us that he would keep getting worse and worse over time, but that at this time, there was no treatment for his particular form of the disease. (If he had been diagnosed with the relapsing remitting form, they might have treated him with one of the various beta-interferon medications, since the beta-interferons were approved for that form only.) The neurologist said he was actually relieved. He had feared that it might be a brain tumor. I felt differently. I felt the diagnosis was worse than a brain tumor because there was no operation to at least try to fix it.

Noel and I had married in 1998, and moved to Ridgewood, New Jersey in 1999. I was determined that Noel would find a neurologist in the United States. I started by driving to several offices and taking their educational materials, to get a feel for their qualifications, history, specialties and patient numbers. (I believed that having more patients was a sign of being a better doctor.) I was disappointed to find that none of them had much information about MS. The literature they did have described the standard medications for MS. It became very clear, very fast, that America did not know of a cure, either.

I finally settled on a local group of neurologists. I called and made an appointment for Noel for July 8, 1999. Noel didn't want to go for the appointment. He said he did not want to make MS the focus of his life. He figured that the neurologist in London knew his stuff and that we just had to accept the truth: There was nothing to be done. Noel could live with that.

It seemed completely futile to him, he told me, to keep asking every doctor the same questions until I found one who would tell me what I wanted to hear: that there was a treatment for his MS. I told him that I just wanted a second opinion. I wanted to fight. He didn't.

I persisted and, to humor me, Noel finally gave in. He eventually agreed that it was probably a good idea to have a neurologist in the US. So we went for the appointment.

I really liked Noel's new neurologist. He was very professional. He explained his impressive credentials and told us about all the meetings he attended with the MS experts of the world to keep him up to date with all the latest MS research. According to him, he was the MS expert. This made me feel safe. He told Noel to start on Avonex, a weekly injection, even though Noel didn't have the kind of MS Avonex was approved for. He felt certain Avonex would slow the progression of Noel's MS. I felt so good leaving his office. At last we were doing something to fight back. Noel was calm and willing to give the shots a try.

Noel started Avonex therapy in July 1999. The shots are intramuscular so the needle is about an inch long. Avonex is a beta-interferon shot, which means it suppresses the immune system. (It is widely believed that MS is a result of an overactive immune system—something I was to learn later was just a theory, and maybe not true at all.)

We were very hopeful that Avonex would help Noel, since clinical studies show that it reduces the relapse rate in 35 percent of patients with MS. It does not stop the progression of MS, or even claim to. And it only slows it down for the lucky ones. I am sure that the neurologist explained all of that, but all I heard was that Avonex slows the progression of MS. I found out much later that Biogen, the makers of Avonex, state that it only works on relapsing remitting MS. As our previous neurologist had told us, it is not recommended for primary progressive MS, Noel's kind of MS. But it was the neurologist's belief (which I appreciated so much at the time) that it was much better to do something instead of nothing. I had no idea what the actual odds of its working were. I knew nothing about the drug other than—in my mind—it was going to work. To keep me optimistic, Biogen sent us monthly newsletters filled with stories about happy MS patients on Avonex.

I offered to administer Noel's shots and he accepted. We picked Saturday night because we were told that he would suffer flu-like symptoms for a day or so after each shot, and that he would have these symptoms for up to nine months.

I remember the first shot. Noel mixed it. I read the pamphlet about ten times. It sounded simple. I had to stick the needle in Noel's thigh muscle. He handed me the needle and I stuck it in, released the shot and pulled it out. I pressed gently on the injection site with a cloth that came as part of the kit, and there was very little blood. It seemed easy enough, but I was relieved to get it over with. That time he didn't feel it.

Every Saturday we alternated between his thighs, although we could have used other muscles. There were times when I hit a vein and his blood spurted everywhere, and other times I hit a nerve and he'd jump his own height. It was always a relief to get the shot over with. As time went on, though, the Saturday night shot became part of our routine.

Initially, the flu-like symptoms were very severe, and for about a year, Noel was feverish every Sunday. But it didn't bother his spirits. He handled the side effects very well, with the help of Tylenol and Advil. But as time went on, his body adjusted, and the flu-like symptoms subsided considerably. He needed the Tylenol and Advil less and less. The mental relief because we were actually doing something was huge for me. Our lives were busy, so we didn't think much about Noel's MS.

Even with Avonex, Noel's MS was progressing. His forty-minute train ride home after work was difficult if he didn't get a seat. I started picking him up at the train station, and I could tell immediately by his gait if he'd gotten a seat or not. I told him he should get a cane, so that people on the train would know he needed a seat. But he refused.

When his walk became very bad, Noel would visit his neurologist, and he'd get steroids, which he loved. They made him feel great, but unfortunately, that effect was always short-lived.

By the time our third daughter, Sara, arrived, Noel's MS was visible all the time because he had developed an obvious foot drop. Everywhere we went, it was much easier for him if he was pushing the stroller. Also, his bladder was starting to weaken. His MS was progressing.

Thank Goodness for the Internet!

Then, two things happened: Noel got a cane, and I got a computer.

In November 2001, I started to seriously research MS on the computer. I started reading and reading. It became an obsession. I hated what I read, because most of it seemed so hopeless. But I couldn't stop.

Initially, the learning curve was steep, because I had to wade through so much medical jargon. But I understood it; I was able to piece it all together somehow. The more I read and understood, the easier it was to read and understand more. I firmly concluded that MS stinks. Plain and simple. MS stinks. I didn't share my obsession with Noel. He knew that I was reading about it, but he wasn't interested in what I was reading. I concluded that he was smart, because why know how awful MS can be when Noel might luck out and have a mild case. The more I read, though, the more I realized that very few people with MS have an easy life. It was clear: MS stinks.

Then came January 2002 and Noel started to slip fast. But because of his unusual brand of positive thinking, he didn't seem to mind, even though he knew he was slipping. For instance, cutting the grass became very difficult for him. He would just stop and rest. But he said that he was mentally prepared for the worst, and wanted to enjoy the fact that, though he stumbled and had to rest a little, he was still able to cut the grass. While I admired his attitude, I didn't accept what seemed to be our fate. I wanted to find something that would help him get better.

Since Noel's MS was progressing, it was obvious the Avonex was not working. I decided to get him a walker, and called the pharmacist I bought Noel's cane from, Town and Country Pharmacy in Ridgewood. John, the pharmacist, answered the phone. I told him that my husband had MS. But before I could get to the part about what kind of walker I should buy, John asked me if I had heard of Low Dose Naltrexone. I had never heard of it.

John told me about a customer and friend of his, Fritz Bell (also known as Mr. Goodshape), who hosted a website at http://goodshape.net. Fritz was married to Polly. Polly had very severe MS. Her MS had been progressing rapidly, but it completely stopped progressing once she started taking LDN two years previously. John told me that he compounded LDN for Polly. And although he confessed that he didn't know a great deal about the drug, he did know that it was a safe bet because it had no known side effects. He told me that LDN was cheap, and that he thought it would be worth a shot for Noel. He told me that Mr. Bell had a lot more information on his website. John explained that Noel might have difficulty getting a prescription for the drug because it was not medically recognized as a treatment for MS. He said that some people who could not persuade their neurologists asked their primary care doctors to prescribe the drug for them off-label, because it was already approved at a much higher dose for heroin addicts. Before I hung up, John told me that if I needed help convincing Noel's neurologist, he was more than willing to help me in any way possible. I decided to investigate LDN.

I couldn't believe what I read. Even for an optimist like me, it sounded too good to be true.

The Goodshape site had a link to the official LDN site, http://www.lowdosenaltrexone.org, the website set up by Dr. David Gluck and his son Joel in 1999, to contain the most up-to-date, official information about Dr. Bihari's work with LDN. After a year or two, realizing that they'd like to have a shorter URL, they adopted http://www.LDNinfo.org/, as well. The sites are identical.

Again, I couldn't believe what I read:

> Clinically the results are strongly suggestive of efficacy. Ninety-eight to 99% of people treated with LDN experience no more disease progression, whether the disease category is relapsing remitting or chronic progressive. Dr. Bihari has more than 70 people with MS in his practice and all are stable over an average of three years. The original patient on LDN for MS, now on it for 17 years, has not had an attack or disease progression for 12 years since the one missed month that led to an attack.
>
> In addition, 2,000 or more people with MS have been prescribed LDN by their family MDs or their neurologists based on what they have read on the LDN website or heard about in Internet chat rooms focused on MS. Many such patients with MS, not under Dr. Bihari's care, use the e-mail link on the LDN website to ask questions. Many prescribing physicians do not generally know about LDN.
>
> Only once has a patient reported disease progression while on LDN. In this case, it showed itself five days after he had started the drug. The onset of the episode had apparently preceded the start of LDN.
>
> In addition to the apparent ability of LDN to stop disease progression, approximately two-thirds of MS patients starting LDN have some symptomatic improvement generally

apparent within the first few days. There are two types of such improvement:

- One is reduction in spasticity when this is present, sometimes allowing easier ambulation when spasticity in the legs has been a prominent element of a patient's difficulty in walking or standing. This is unlikely to represent a direct effect of LDN on the disease process, but rather reduction in the irritability in nervous tissue surrounding plaques. Endorphins have been shown to reduce irritability of nervous tissue, e.g., by reducing seizures in patients with epilepsy.

- The other area of symptomatic improvement in some patients is a reduction in MS-related fatigue. This is, also, not likely due to a direct effect on the MS disease process, but rather an indirect one caused by restoration of normal endorphin levels improving energy.

Patients who are in the midst of an acute exacerbation when they start LDN have generally shown rapid resolution of the attack. In two patients, chronic visual impairment due to old episodes of optic neuritis has shown fluctuating improvement.

It should be emphasized that in spite of the plentitude of clinical experience described above, in the absence of a formal clinical trial of LDN in MS, these results cannot be considered scientific, but rather anecdotal. A clinical trial, preferably by a pharmaceutical company with some experience with MS, is clearly needed to determine whether these results can be replicated. If they can be, they are likely to lead to widespread use of this extremely non-toxic drug in the treatment of MS.

—From http://www.lowdosenaltrexone.org/ldn_and_ms.htm

That was my starting point.

At that time, I was well aware of the chances of the standard MS drugs slowing the progression of relapsing remitting MS only, but none of them came remotely close to what I was reading about LDN. This was saying that LDN does not slow the progression; it actually stops the progression 98 to 99 percent of the time, regardless of the type of MS. It was unbelievable.

I decided that I didn't want to know anything more about LDN until I thoroughly investigated the doctor behind these claims, Dr. Bernard Bihari. I also wanted to quickly figure out who was profiting from the website that was advertising these bold claims.

I performed an Internet search on Dr. Bernard Bihari, which led me to the home page of the LDN web site that was linked to Goodshape's site. I laughed because it took me a while to travel that circle. I noticed that Dr. Bihari's curriculum vitae (CV) was part of the site. It said that he got his MD degree from Harvard and listed his New York State Medical License number: 088158. I used that number to verify part of his CV with the New York State Education Department. I found his record. He was one hundred percent what he said he was.

I continued to investigate and read on his CV that he was board certified since 1970. I confirmed that information with the American Board of Psychiatry and Neurology. His CV also stated that he was an attending physician at Beth Israel Medical Center in New York, so I phoned Beth Israel and confirmed that information. I concluded that it was difficult to believe that Dr. Bihari was a quack because his credentials were solid.

Then I checked out the website itself to see who was sponsoring it. I was again impressed to learn that it was a nonprofit website:

> This website is sponsored by Advocates for Therapeutic Immunology. The purpose of this website is to provide information to patients and physicians about important therapeutic breakthroughs in advanced medical immunology. The authors of this site do not profit from the sale of LDN or from website traffic, and are in no way associated with any pharmaceutical manufacturer or pharmacy.

I became convinced that Dr. Bihari was not a quack and was not trying to make a fast dollar. I was intrigued, to say the least. Next, I decided to find out what LDN actually was.

I learned that LDN stood for Low Dose Naltrexone. Naltrexone hydrochloride is a white powder chemical compound. It is a drug that is listed in the *Physicians' Desk Reference*® (*PDR*), and is an approved treatment for substance abuse, such as heroin addiction. Since it is listed in the *PDR*, doctors may use their own judgment in deciding whether to prescribe naltrexone off-label to other individuals, such as those with MS and other autoimmune diseases.

Naltrexone is marketed in generic form, naltrexone hydrochloride, under the trade names Revia, Nodict, Vivtrol and Depade. Although it is primarily a narcotic antagonist, which means it counteracts the effects of narcotics, it has also been shown to reduce craving and consumption for some patients who are alcohol-dependent. The FDA-approved standard dose given to patients with a substance abuse problem is 50 mg.

At first I didn't understand how a drug used for substance abuse could help people with MS. Then I learned that naltrexone in different doses does completely different things. At a low dose of 4.5 mg, Dr. Bihari was using LDN to boost the immune systems of his patients. I learned that such thinking flies in the face of conventional MS thinking, because the standard MS medications work on suppressing the immune system based on the theory that people with MS have an overactive immune system. Dr. Bihari was challenging all conventional views of MS by trying to boost the immune system, as opposed to suppressing it. I liked that because I had seen conventional medicine fail Noel.

So, how does LDN actually work? Imagine you are a heroin addict. You want to get over your addiction, so you take the FDA-approved 50 mg naltrexone daily. Some addicts actually take up to 200 mg daily. Then you have a weak moment and decide to take a hit of heroin. Despite the hit, you won't get high, because at 50 mg, naltrexone will block the opioid receptors in your brain for twenty-four hours. It is hoped that an addict will stop taking the heroin once he or she sees that the naltrexone prevents the expected high.

Interestingly, naltrexone acts very differently at high doses than it does at low doses. At a low dose of 4.5 mg, naltrexone blocks the same opioid receptors, but only for three or four hours. During that time, the pituitary and adrenal glands respond to the inability of those receptors to produce endorphins, and after that time, flood the body with three times more endorphins than usual. Although the short blockade ends, the increased endorphins last most of the day and boost the immune system enough to ensure that it stops attacking one's own tissues. That is why it works for such a wide range of autoimmune diseases.

But, there is a huge difference between the actions of high-dose and low-dose naltrexone. So, there are a few things you must know if you are a drug or alcohol addict, and also have a condition based on a disturbed immune system, like MS. If you take the FDA-approved 50 mg naltrexone (or higher) for your addiction, your MS will actually get worse, because you are blocking endorphin reception for too long a period of time. You see, at high doses, naltrexone will not rectify a disturbed immune system. Therefore, in this instance, it would be wise to avoid taking naltrexone at 50 mg or higher.

Similarly, if you have both a drug or alcohol problem and cancer, it would not be wise to take naltrexone, either. In high doses, naltrexone also stimulates cancer progression. So, again, while the high dose of naltrexone would counter your drug or alcohol addiction, your cancer would actually get worse. There is no point in curing an addiction, and then dying of cancer, or having your autoimmune condition progress. This piece of important information—that, in high doses (at the FDA-approved dose) naltrexone stimulates both cancer and autoimmune disease progression—was not picked up in the FDA trials that approved naltrexone for various addictions.

Even worse, ironically, naltrexone, at the dose at which it was approved by the FDA, has failed miserably over time with actual patients. The reason: It blocks endorphin production for too long a period of time, which induces severe depression in most cases. So, sadly, naltrexone is recognized by doctors (and in their "bible," the *Physicians' Desk Reference*) for conditions for which it is not really effective, while it has an amazing potential in much lower doses for a myriad of other conditions. Unfortunately, most doctors don't know about these other uses.

Many people ask why, if LDN is so effective for these other conditions, studies are not conducted to prove this. The truth is that, once a drug has been FDA-approved at any dose—and especially when it is no longer under patent, and is thus, a generic—it is very difficult to get funding for further testing. Why? Because it will no longer bring any company a lot of money.

I was curious as to what prompted Dr. Bihari's use of LDN, so I read more and dug deeper. I learned that Dr. Bihari's early work consisted of helping those afflicted with drug and alcohol abuse in New York City. From there, in the 1980s, his work extended to the HIV and AIDS community. It was during this time, after years of experimenting with naltrexone dosing, that he discovered the therapeutic effects of LDN for HIV and AIDS. He observed that addicts with HIV did not develop full-blown AIDS when they took a low dose of naltrexone. From what I know of the man, I believe that his heart lay in helping the AIDS epidemic, and that he stumbled into helping the MS community serendipitously.

In 1988, his daughter's best friend, Chris Lombardi, was diagnosed with MS. Because Dr. Bihari had seen the capability of LDN to boost the immune system in his HIV and AIDS patients, he prescribed LDN for Chris. He believed that HIV and AIDS and MS had one thing in common: They were diseases based on disturbed immune systems. So, it was more than plausible, in Dr. Bihari's mind, that LDN would work for MS, seeing as it was showing great promise in HIV and AIDS patients in his practice.

Chris was 22 in 1988 and no approved treatment for MS existed at that time. Dr. Bihari prescribed 3 mg LDN. She took it for five years with no progression of her disease. Then, she went out of state and her LDN supply ran out. She felt so good that she figured she didn't need LDN anymore. So she stopped taking it. Within a month, her MS started to flare up again. She immediately resumed LDN treatment. Chris was the first MS patient on LDN; she is a remarkable testimony to its benefits.

For many years since 1988, Dr. Bihari dedicated himself to the AIDS crisis, but through word of mouth, LDN's potential for MS spread, and he was contacted—though slowly at first—by more and more people suffering with MS. By the time I actually followed his story through and picked up the phone to speak with him, he had fewer than eighty patients with MS. But they were all stable, regardless of the type of MS they were diagnosed with.

When I finally got up the nerve to call Dr. Bihari—his address and phone number were part of his CV that was posted on the LDN site—Noel was at work and my three girls were napping. I had no idea what to expect, but I was more than pleasantly surprised.

My first surprise was that Dr. Bihari actually answered the phone himself. I introduced myself and explained that I had been reading about his work on the Internet and wanted to talk to him about it before presenting it all to Noel. Dr. Bihari was very friendly. I was honest with him and told him that LDN sounded too good to be true. I explained that I didn't want to play on Noel's emotions and I couldn't trust my own. I had to be very certain of my information before I even thought about raising Noel's hopes.

Dr. Bihari completely understood and proceeded to assure me that everything I had read about LDN was true. He started at the very beginning and explained everything to me in terms I could understand. His manner was very relaxed. He was easy to talk with and listen to. I felt his compassion. He told me about his work with the AIDS and HIV community, but I wasn't interested in any of that at the time. I just wanted to know about LDN and MS.

Dr. Bihari told me that he believed everybody with an autoimmune disorder has low levels of endorphins. Before he explained what endorphins were, he told me exactly what an autoimmune disease is. He said that the word "auto" is the Greek word for self. The immune system is a complicated network that normally works to defend the body and eliminate infections. But if a person has an autoimmune disease, the immune system mistakenly attacks itself, targeting the cells, tissues and organs of a person's own body. There are many different autoimmune diseases, and they can each affect the body in different ways. For example, the autoimmune reaction is directed against the brain and spinal cord in multiple sclerosis, and against the gut in Crohn's disease.

I had read on the Internet that there are many theories as to what MS actually is, and it is even debated as to whether or not it is autoimmune. Also, the definitions and naming of various types and stages of MS are highly debated. Everything about MS is debated. It is incredibly elusive. That is what makes it even more frustrating, but Dr. Bihari firmly believes that MS is an autoimmune disease. He believes that is why LDN stops it in its tracks.

Dr. Bihari explained that just as the sex hormone, testosterone, controls sexual function, endorphins control and regulate the immune system. He said he believes that endorphin production has a biological clock, which people call a circadian rhythm, and that that internal human biological clock dictates that most of our endorphins are produced nightly. He calculated that the best time to take LDN would be between 9:00 p.m. and 2:00 a.m. He said that LDN, if taken nightly, causes endorphin production to triple, bringing the levels up to normal, and once normal, the immune system stops attacking itself. Dr. Bihari claims that if endorphin production is regulated, the endorphins will be able to control and regulate the immune system. Hence, the immune system will no longer attack itself. He told me that was why none of his MS patients had progressed. It was that simple.

"LDN is not a cure for MS," he insisted. He stated that LDN would only remove the last three months of damage, if Noel was lucky. But it seemed to be universal in stopping MS disease progression.

That day, I spoke with Dr. Bihari for nearly an hour. Before hanging up, I offered to pay him, but he refused. He said he was delighted I had found the LDN website, and that he was sure it would help Noel. He explained that any doctor could prescribe LDN off-label for his or her patients, and added that, if Noel's neurologist or general doctor wanted to speak with him, he would be glad to share his case studies. He also told me that, if Noel decided to take LDN, we should be sure it was compounded as described on the LDN website.

Many years have passed since that phone call.

Before making my final decision to present this information about LDN to Noel, I checked out a few of the online message boards. While there are several today, back then there were only a few message boards: Goodshape's, and one or two others. I started by "lurking" on the Goodshape message board. Then I joined in the discussions there. Several people told of their success with LDN. But they also warned me of potential nightmare dealings with neurologists and doctors, in general, but also assured me that the fight would be worth it in the end. Their assertion that LDN is the best possible treatment for MS was always the bottom line. They insisted that I never give up.

I dug some more because I could not help but think that if LDN was so great, then why on earth was it such a secret? I questioned why Noel's neurologist didn't know about it. After all, he attended most of the MS meetings in New York along with the best MS experts in the world. It seemed logical to assume that if there was anything worth knowing about LDN, then he would know about it. I deduced that if Noel's neurologist knew about LDN, then Noel would have been on it. So I figured that Noel's neurologist was not aware of LDN and if he was aware of it, then it was obvious that he was not convinced of its merits.

I also questioned why in the world nothing was published about LDN and MS. But, at that time, I didn't yet understand the mechanics of publishing in the medical world. I could only assume that it is not very easy for a cheap, generic drug with no side effects and such amazing promise to get published. It was evident that I had more loose ends to tie up before sharing my findings with family and friends, because I knew that I had to be prepared to answer their obvious questions.

I posted my concerns on Goodshape's site. And the replies came in. The reason LDN has not hit the masses is because the drug companies dishing out the expensive drugs to MS patients stand to lose far too much money. It was spelled out to me that pharmaceutical companies make a nice profit tending to MS victims and that they were acting behind the scenes in their own best interests. The people on the message board strongly implied that the MS drug companies were actively preventing LDN from reaching the masses. Granted, MS therapies are expensive, and hence, lucrative. The plot started to thicken and my blood started to boil. Initially, I refused to believe that the world was so corrupt. I refused to believe what I read. Part of me still does. A big part of me still cannot buy into the theory, now believed by many to be true. Though Avonex costs $2,000 a month, compared to approximately $35 a month for LDN, I still couldn't buy into this theory because I felt that it was based on paranoia. Maybe at first I believed it, because

I wanted somebody to blame. But as soon as I thought about it in depth, I rejected it. Now, I am not so sure.

But I started to understand why Dr. Bihari had problems getting the drug into a scientific trial in the US. It made business sense to me. LDN is a cheap generic drug. It is already FDA-approved at ten times the dose used for autoimmune diseases, so it holds no monetary incentive for any pharmaceutical company, or US government body, to run a series of expensive trials. Because it is generic, it means that anybody can sell it and anyone can buy it. Actually, the US government would save millions of dollars in the long run if even one-tenth of what Dr. Bihari claims to be true is, in fact, true—because more people would be able to work and require less financial support from the state. Corporate America, however, has a short-term view of profit and works against the potential of a cheap drug, despite the hope it holds for its citizens. That is the sad and tragic reality. But, are the big, bad, profit-crazy drug companies actually actively stopping LDN getting out there? I didn't and still don't believe that.

The problem I have with that theory is that the LDN community is too small. We are not big or scary enough yet to make any drug company take us seriously. But our community is now getting bigger, and maybe the pharmaceutical companies are afraid of what would happen if more people knew about LDN.

But, as far as I could see, in 2002, there were a handful of LDN advocates who saw LDN work. MS, however, is very elusive, so the same number of people could just as easily have been saying that the best way to stop MS progression is to pat your head and rub your tummy three times daily. The enigmatic world of MS provides a fertile breeding ground for quackery.

With regard to reaching the masses with LDN, though, I firmly believe that there is no bad guy actively trying to prevent it from happening. I can see how the good guys, such as the MS societies, whose duty it is to help people with MS, could be perceived as the bad guys simply because they openly want as little as possible to do with LDN. However, I believe that the real problem with getting anybody to seriously investigate the potential of LDN, particularly in the US, comes down to two major things. It lacks financial incentive and equally, it lacks credibility. It is too simple a theory—almost too ridiculous to believe. I mean, even to me, an optimist by nature, with my back against the wall, it was unbelievable.

When I look at the situation in Ireland, I see that the government pays for all of the expensive MS medications for each person who decides to take them. In Ireland, 6,000 people have MS, and about 2,000 of them use a standard MS therapy. Anybody can do the math: 1,200 euros a month per person for the standard MS drugs, versus 30 euros a month for LDN. Of course, one would think that the Irish government would prefer to pay for the LDN—because it's cheaper, and because, with it, fewer people would be financially dependent on the government because of disability. In 2004, Dr. Bihari presented the Irish government with a proposal to do a trial on LDN for MS. But the Irish government turned his proposal down. (Editor's note: For the full text, see the Appendix.) The only reason I can think of for why they did this is because of credibility. I think they simply couldn't believe that what we say about LDN is true. (However, a skeptic would question whether or not the government is in bed with the pharmaceutical companies.)

Also, for a funder to conduct an LDN trial requires a leap of faith, because the whole theory of how LDN works flies in the face of conventional thinking. As Dr. Bihari pointed out to me, conventional thinking states that to treat an autoimmune disease, you must suppress the immune system. Therefore, billions of dollars have been spent on producing highly toxic, expensive and ineffective medications that reflect this theory. And doctors are used to prescribing these drugs, even though they see that many patients don't respond well to them.

Again, as Dr. Bihari pointed out to me, LDN works by mobilizing the body's natural defense system and regulating our own immune system, so that our immune system can fight the disease. The theory is beautiful, almost poetic, and highly supported by patient-based evidence and clinical medicine. But pharmaceutical companies and governments don't want to risk funding an actual trial, despite the potential it holds for future monetary savings, not to mention future lives.

Also, the fact that it works for so many illnesses sounds "too good to be true" to many scientists. But all of these illnesses that LDN helps have something in common: a compromised immune system.

It is such a shame that people don't seem to believe us that LDN works so well for so many conditions. Think how much money our governments could save.

By August 2002, I had reached a point where I felt that I had thoroughly investigated LDN, and I decided it was time to present my findings to Noel.

Frankly, it wasn't easy. Even though I had done what I knew was some really impressive research, Noel was skeptical. When I told him about my conversations with my "virtual friends" in cyberspace, I could tell that he thought I'd lost my mind. I expected that. Then I told him about my conversation with Dr. Bihari. Noel said that if there was any truth in what I was saying, then his neurologist would know about LDN. I explained to him that it was quite possible that his neurologist would not know about it, since LDN was relatively new at that time, and wasn't "clinically proven." But since it was cheap and without side effects, I thought he should try it.

Noel didn't agree. But I pushed. Finally, Noel said he wanted to try one more blast of steroids. But he said I could come with him to his next neurologist's appointment to try to convince the doctor to prescribe LDN. I agreed.

Our visit with the neurologist went as I expected it would, with his neurologist telling me of all the MS meetings he attended. He told me that LDN had not gone through any scientific trial, and that if there was anything at all worth knowing about LDN, then he certainly would know about it. I asked him if LDN could possibly do Noel any harm. He shrugged and said he couldn't see any. I think to humor me—and to get rid of me—the neurologist finally wrote Noel a script (prescription) for 3 mg of LDN. He also wrote a script for Copaxone, even though we all knew that Copaxone was not supposed to have any benefit for Noel's kind of MS, PPMS. Copaxone has only been tested for relapsing remitting MS (RRMS), which Noel doesn't have. And, of course, Noel got his prescription for steroids.

That was on September 11, 2002. Noel started taking LDN the next day.

The immediate improvements were stark. It was incredible. Within six weeks, Noel's bladder had greatly improved, and he stopped falling over. Although he still needed his cane around the house, he was able to take six or seven steps without it. There were definite improvements, but the most amazing thing for me was that the onslaught of the disease had finally stopped. Noel's MS had stopped progressing. Could our nightmare really be over? For the first time ever, I felt that his MS was under arrest. There is nothing better than the release from the onslaught of a progressive degenerative disease. As always, Noel remained calm. He didn't get overly excited because mentally he did not buy into it at all. He couldn't afford to do that. But our family and friends could not believe the visible improvement in him. These were happy days.

As January 2003 passed, I became more and more convinced that LDN was working. Noel was, without question, stable. He no longer had to heave himself off the couch, and for the first time in about ten years, his feet were warm again. His complexion was also much better. I remember thinking that he just looked healthy. The biggest benefit, of course, was that the onslaught had stopped. And now, seven years later, his MS has still not progressed at all since then.

I am now a staunch and very vocal LDN advocate. Many other family members and friends have gone on LDN because of me; I am active in the LDN community. In 2005, *Up the Creek With a Paddle*, my book about our family's experiences with LDN, was published; a second edition came out in 2009. And in 2009, too, I began my Internet radio show on blogtalkradio. (http://www.blogtalkradio.com/mary-boyle-bradley/) On my show, I have interviewed doctors and patients alike from the US and from the British Isles. Doctors include Dr. David Gluck, Dr. Tom Gilhooly, Dr. Phil Boyle (my brother), Dr. Ian Zagon, Dr. Burt Berkson and Dr. Skip Lenz (a compounding pharmacist). Among the patient advocates I have interviewed: Jayne Crocker and Andrew Barnett, Vicky Finlayson, Linda Elsegood, SammyJo Wilkinson, Aletha Whitmann and Joe Wouk. The list goes on. I will not stop talking about LDN, and promoting it, until I am convinced that every single person who needs to know about LDN knows about it. My aim—and the aim of all the other LDN advocates—is that LDN will be available to everyone who needs it as a first-line treatment, rather than as a last resort that is stumbled upon, almost by accident.

I urge you to listen to Mary's interviews on blogtalkradio: http://www.blogtalkradio.com/mary-boyle-bradley. While she is not currently conducting interviews, you can learn a lot more about LDN by listening to those that are online.

CHAPTER 14

Malcolm West on LDN

"A Cash Cow No More!"

I first met Malcolm West while talking (via Skype) with other LDN advocates (Linda Elsegood and SammyJo Wilkinson) in August 2009. We were strategizing about how to get the word out about the first International LDN Awareness Week the following October (2010). When I heard Malcolm's story, I knew he had to write a chapter for my book, because his story struck a very special chord with me.

The reason I found his story so compelling is that, as long as Malcolm was "rich"—i.e., with a well-paying job and "Cadillac health insurance"—he was able to afford the expensive, toxic, and (for him) ineffective MS drugs that are the standard of care. But, he was also at the behest of the conventional medical system. It was only when he lost his job—and with it, his health insurance—and could no longer afford the treatments his doctors had been prescribing that he was left to his own devices. It was up to him to find an inexpensive treatment for his MS. He found LDN, and he hasn't looked back.

As you will see, Malcolm makes a really strong argument for using LDN first, before too much time has elapsed, and before one's MS (or other autoimmune disease) has progressed. Malcolm believes that, had he found LDN sooner, he would not have any of the pre-LDN disabilities he now has. He is working hard so that others will find LDN earlier than he did.

In 1991, shortly after the birth of my son, I began losing my balance and stumbling into things. I was 34, in good health, a competitive squash and soccer player. What was going on with me? Was it the stress of our first child? Was it the stress of my job? I called my doctor, who sent me to an ear, nose and throat specialist, who performed many tests, but found nothing. Was it a brain tumor? Next, I was referred to a top neurologist at Georgetown University Hospital, who did more tests. But unfortunately, still no answers. I was put on a drug called Tegretol for the control of seizures. Since I did not have seizures, I'm not sure why I was prescribed Tegretol. But I was.

After a month or so, my condition got a little better, except for an annoying tingling and numbness in my feet, weakness in my left arm and tightness around my rib cage. I hoped that these symptoms would go away; I just tried to ignore them.

Two years later, my symptoms increased to having double vision and trouble focusing. When I turned to the left, my right eye wouldn't follow my left eye. I went back to the doctor, and to another neurologist. Again, more tests. This neurologist thought it was probably multiple sclerosis (MS). I knew nothing about MS. In about two weeks, after a five-day home infusion of steroids, my vision returned to normal. But the strange symptoms persisted, coming and going, some old, some new. Then, I had another attack of optic neuritis, and was again prescribed home steroids. My balance got worse, and because I wasn't able to lift my left foot properly, I started tripping. My squash and soccer days were over. Besides, now we had a new baby girl, and there was no time for games anyway.

At about this time, a new drug was approved for MS, a betainterferon called Avonex, made by the Biogen Corporation. I had to wait a year until enough of it became available, but finally I was able to get it. Avonex requires a weekly intramuscular injection with a two-inch needle. The side effects made me feel like I was coming down with the flu during the twelve hours following each injection. Another side effect was ongoing depression. Because of Avonex's toxicity, I had to get blood tests every three months to make sure it wasn't damaging my liver. For the next five years, my wife and I faithfully injected this drug into my arms or legs every Saturday night. The intramuscular shot was difficult for me to do by myself, so my wife helped, which she hated. Sometimes we would hit a vein, or a bone. When we hit a vein, the drug went directly into my bloodstream and soon caused uncontrollable shaking. Every Sunday, I felt sick. Even with these weekly injections, my MS symptoms continued to slowly progress.

My limp was now becoming more apparent to everyone. I tired easily and couldn't walk long distances without the help of a cane. People at work started asking me what was wrong and I could no longer brush them off with an excuse. I started to confide in some of my closest co-workers about my MS. Many of them didn't know how to respond, since they had only heard scary things about MS, about crippled, unfortunate people confined to wheelchairs, even bedridden.

My new neurologist decided that Avonex was no longer working and switched me over to a new, more powerful interferon drug, Rebif. Rebif involved three weekly injections.

But it didn't help, either. The flu-like side effects persisted, and after two years, the depression became unbearable. My neurologist suggested adding an anti-depressant drug or trying another new MS drug, Copaxone, a once-a-day shot. While the Copaxone involved a smaller needle and the shots often bruised or left welts on my body, I was no longer feeling sick and depressed. I continued with Copaxone for two more years. But still, my MS continued to progress. Soon I could no longer walk more than ten feet without a walker. I bought a wheelchair and an electric scooter.

My neurologist now decided that the Copaxone was no longer working, either. I asked him about a drug I had recently read about on the Internet called Low Dose Naltrexone (LDN). He quickly dismissed me, saying there was no clinical data on LDN. It was, he said, an "Internet cult drug." I asked him questions about how LDN works, but it was obvious that he knew nothing about it. Nor was he willing to learn about it, or talk with me about it. Instead, he recommended that, since the drugs I had tried so far weren't working, I begin chemotherapy treatment. (Editor's note: In a further effort to suppress the immune system, chemotherapy is sometimes given to MS patients when the more-often-prescribed drugs haven't worked. The primary function of all of these standard-of-care MS drugs and treatments is to suppress the immune system.)

For the next year—this was 2004—every three months, I went to an infusion center where they injected a dark, inky blue chemo into my veins. I began losing my hair, was nauseous for several days, constipated and urinated blue. It was obvious that this drug was especially toxic because before each session I had to get an $1,800 test at the hospital to make sure the chemo was not permanently damaging my heart function. For the chemo, they injected radioactive dye into my bloodstream. The technicians wore gloves to protect themselves from any exposure. My blood was also tested before every infusion for the possibility of developing leukemia.

In 2004, another new MS drug was approved: Tysabri, a monoclonal antibody, a drug that prevents T-cells from crossing the blood-brain barrier and attacking the myelin nerve coating. Tysabri involved an infusion every four weeks at a cost of over $4,000 each time. I was referred to a new neurologist for a second opinion. He authorized the drug and my health insurance approved it. With Tysabri, I would have to have a $2,000 MRI scan every six months because this drug can cause Progressive Multifocal Leukoencephalitis (PML), a rare and usually fatal viral disease characterized by progressive damage to the white matter in your brain. People with compromised immune systems get PML, so people with MS are particularly susceptible. Interferons, chemotherapy and Tysabri all suppress the immune system. Biogen, the company that makes Tysabri, originally conducted trials on Tysabri, in combination with their interferon drug, Avonex, hoping for better results and profit potential. The combination proved too much for several MS patients, who developed PML and died. Several others sustained permanent brain damage. Biogen briefly withdrew Tysabri from the market, but reintroduced it in late 2005 as a monotherapy with an FDA "black box" warning. (Editor's note: A "black box" warning is a type of warning that the FDA requires a pharmaceutical company to include in the package inserts of certain drugs. It signifies that "medical studies indicate that the drug carries a significant risk of serious or even life-threatening adverse effects." "Black box" itself refers to the fact that this warning is surrounded by a "black box," so that it will stand out: http://en.wikipedia.org/wiki/Black_box_warning.)

Even though I wasn't getting any better, and even though I was wary of taking this drug, I was grateful to have good health insurance because my MS treatments, which were always expensive, were now costing well over $40,000 a year.

Every four weeks, my wife drove me to the infusion center where I shared the room with approximately twelve other patients, most of whom were receiving chemotherapy for some type of cancer. I felt strangely fortunate that I "only" had MS. On the other hand, I felt unfortunate to be the only one who usually arrived in a wheelchair. At the infusion center, when people completed their chemo treatments they rang a bell on the wall and the nurses all cheered and wished them good luck. There was always a cake and lots of food and snacks available, supplied free by a constant stream of attractive pharmaceutical sales representatives. As time passed, my wife and I became very disappointed with Tysabri, since it turned out not to be the miracle drug some people reported. There seemed to be no end to this treatment, and I never got to ring the bell. (Editor's note: The ringing of the bell at the completion of chemotherapy treatment did not mean that the patient had gotten better. It just meant that the patient had gone through the prescribed number of treatments. Those treatments may—or may not—have stopped the patient's cancer. His or her doctor would evaluate this later, and decide whether further treatment was needed.)

Because I could no longer walk and travel on company business, I lost my job in the beginning of 2008. The human resources manager told me they were simply downsizing as a result of the weak economy, and unfortunately, there were no other positions appropriate for me, that the company was struggling. But we both knew I was let go because I was now in a wheelchair. Discrimination can be hard to prove in a recession.

No job meant that soon there would be no more health insurance for my family. I contacted my health insurance provider to inquire how much the new monthly premium would cost after COBRA expired. I was told the premium would double from $1,486 to approximately $3,000 a month. While under the law, this health insurance company had to accept me regardless of having MS as a preexisting condition, other insurance providers would not have the same obligation. My wife and I decided to drop health insurance coverage for ourselves after COBRA expired, and just buy HMO policies for the children.

At this point, I decided to start my own business, working from home creating websites for meetings and events, even though it was not the best time to start such a business. The Great Recession was tough on everyone. After eighteen infusions of Tysabri, I decided it was time to stop. Now that COBRA had expired, we could not afford the $4,000 monthly cost of treatment on our own. And Tysabri didn't seem to be working for me anyway. Besides, I knew that the longer you take it, the greater your risk for developing PML. It is known that one out of every 1,000 Tysabri users develops PML. As of October 2009, twenty-three people had developed the brain infection. (http://www.xconomy.com/boston/2009/10/23/biogen-shares-drop-as-tysabri-pml-cases-climb-to-23-europe-may-seek-drug-holiday/) And as of November 2, 2010, according to the MS Society, the number had risen to seventy-five confirmed cases. As of September 2010, 75,500 people worldwide have used the drug. (http://www.nationalmssociety.org/news/news-detail/index.aspx?nid=2308) Biogen still recommends MRIs every six months to check for PML infection.

While all MS drug costs have increased dramatically over the past five years, Tysabri only increased 5.8 percent in 2009. And while Avonex increased 9 percent in 2009, it has actually increased in price 53 percent since 2007. A July 17, 2009 article in *The Wall Street Journal* noted that Biogen has been able to raise prices in the middle of a recession, and that the company has embarked on a new effort to persuade doctors and patients that Tysabri's potential PML side effect is minimal: http://online.wsj.com/article/SB124774457299150965.html.

Now with no health insurance, I turned my attention back to Low Dose Naltrexone (LDN), which I knew was inexpensive. Besides LDN, I really had no options for treating my MS other than begging for financial assistance from Biogen, or from one of the other MS drug companies. However, in order to qualify for assistance, we would first have to drain our savings and our children's college fund.

To this day, we continue to receive the glossy direct mailers from Biogen touting the many benefits of Tysabri therapy. They show attractive, happy MS patients leading active lives, thanks to Tysabri. In these brochures, no one is using a cane, a walker, an electric scooter or a wheelchair. There are no disabled people in any MS drug advertisements, only attractive, healthy people smiling, laughing, walking, running, climbing and biking. Having MS almost looks like fun. And just about every MS drug company has a celebrity spokesperson who claims their drug contributes to their active, productive life.

Soon after I stopped taking Tysabri, a woman from Biogen called me to ask why I had stopped. Was there a problem? How could she help?

At this point, again, I asked my neurologist to write me a prescription for LDN and again, he declined. Instead, he recommended I undergo plasmapherisis, a process where they admit you to the hospital and your blood is removed. The plasma is then separated from the blood cells, and the blood cells are returned with a saline solution, evidently free of the cells that were attacking your myelin. My doctor told me that, although he couldn't guarantee that it would stop my MS progression, he thought it was worth trying. I told him I'd consider it. (I had no idea how I would even pay for it.) I left his office, never to return.

Thank Goodness for the Internet!

The Internet is a gift for people with MS. Until about five to six years ago, the only way you could share information with other multiple sclerosis patients was by going to a monthly National Multiple Sclerosis Society meeting or attending a drug company-sponsored seminar. There, a neurologist would give a talk about new MS drug treatments, while you'd be served a hotel chicken dinner. You'd leave with a new tote bag bearing the drug company's logo, and brochures and pens, handed out by attractive drug company sales representatives. Of course, they'd get your name and address and soon you'd begin receiving direct mailers with pictures of happy people enjoying an active MS lifestyle while taking their company's drug. The neurologist would leave with new patient referrals and a speaking fee from the drug company sponsor.

Now, MS patients can communicate worldwide through many websites and discussion forums. Soon, I found out more about Low Dose Naltrexone and was referred to a doctor who agreed to prescribe it with only a phone appointment. He didn't accept health insurance, which was fine, since I didn't have any. His charge for the appointment was very affordable for me: $135.

When I called this doctor and asked him what he thought of LDN, his words were direct: "LDN stops MS in its tracks." He wrote me a prescription for a three-month supply and I filled it by mail order at a compounding pharmacy in Florida for $55. The doctor would have to renew my prescription every three months, at a cost to me of $35 a month.

Excited, I took my first 1.5 mg LDN capsule and went to bed. A night of interrupted sleep and vivid dreams followed, but the next day I awoke with a smile on my face. The resulting 200 to 300 percent increase in endorphin production from LDN caused me to feel pretty good. After a few more nights, the disturbed sleep patterns started to dissipate, though my dreams continued to be vivid and entertaining.

After two weeks, I doubled my dosage of LDN to 3 mg, as instructed. In another two weeks, I increased it to 4.5 mg, the recommended dose for multiple sclerosis and other autoimmune diseases. While I experienced some stiffness in my legs, I soon found that the drug caused no other side effects, besides deep dreams and perhaps the most restful sleep I had experienced in decades.

My multiple sclerosis fatigue lifted almost immediately. Prior to taking LDN, it was not uncommon for me to have to take a nap two or three times a day. People who have MS often complain that fatigue is the most difficult symptom they struggle with, and many take additional drugs to help them stay awake. My balance also improved and I found myself not falling as much as I made my way through the house with my cane or walker. My vision, which often suffered from optic neuritis, the result of MS plaque on my optic nerve, returned to normal.

One problem almost all people with multiple sclerosis have is the urinary urgency or incontinence, and I was no exception. Since starting LDN, rushed visits to the bathroom have diminished greatly. Finally, my general mood became more elevated. I felt great. No more depression side effects, like I had experienced while on the interferon treatments. And it was a cheap little pill! No shots. No infusions. No blood tests. No heart scans. No neurologists. My MS drug therapy was now costing me less than $500 a year.

Yet, most important—and most exciting—is that after taking Low Dose Naltrexone now for over a year, my MS does not seem to be getting any worse. At best, the FDA-approved multiple sclerosis drugs have only been found in clinical trials to slow progression between 30 and 40 percent. The most toxic and invasive treatment, Tysabri, has been shown to be 66 percent effective in slowing progression with multiple sclerosis patients who have the relapsing remitting form of the disease. People usually start by taking an interferon treatment first, and if that fails to slow progression, a neurologist will recommend Tysabri.

All these treatments are very expensive, costing between $2,000 and $4,000 per month. The accompanying tests—such as MRIs and blood tests—and doctors' visits are extra. All have significant toxic side effects and severely compromise the body's immune system. All multiple sclerosis drug treatments are based on the assumption that the way to treat the disease is to suppress the immune system. The common belief is that rogue T-cells are for some reason attacking the myelin coating of nerves in the brain and spinal cord. Preventing these T-cells from attacking the myelin is the primary function of all MS drugs. Likewise, other autoimmune disease treatments such as rheumatoid arthritis, fibromyalgia, lupus and Crohn's disease are based on the same assumption: Suppress the immune system.

Running contrary to this assumption, LDN boosts the body's endorphin production the day after you take it, and these increased endorphins better regulate the immune system. Other substances, like vitamin D and omega-3 fatty acids, also help regulate the immune system. As the human body ages, its capability to effectively produce endorphins declines. As a result, the immune system weakens and becomes less capable of protecting us from illness, chronic diseases and cancer.

It is well known that multiple sclerosis is largely a Western disease. People usually come down with MS in adulthood and most often, these people live in regions of the world that receive less sunlight. Or they may pursue a lifestyle that limits their exposure to sunlight. Or they eat a fatty diet that is not rich in omega-3 fatty acids. Or they may have been exposed to some type of environmental toxicity. These lifestyle issues, coupled with possible genetic factors, appear to make some individuals more prone to developing multiple sclerosis, as well as other similar autoimmune diseases. People with MS are almost always found to have low vitamin D levels and, accordingly, low endorphin levels.

Further supporting these findings would be the evidence that many people with multiple sclerosis report success in limiting disease progression by regular exercise and following a low-fat diet rich in omega-3 nutrients. These people are increasing endorphin production and maintaining a well-regulated immune system. LDN basically does the same thing. The limited dose of naltrexone taken at bedtime blocks opioid receptors and tricks the pituitary gland into over-producing endorphins. In the next sixteen hours, the pituitary gland pumps out 200-300 percent of the normal amount of endorphins. Taking LDN is essentially like going for a run every day without your muscles participating. For people with a chronic disease like MS, which limits mobility, LDN may be the only way to consistently generate sufficient endorphins to regulate the immune system. The implications of maintaining high endorphin production as the body ages are profound. We already know that older people who incorporate exercise into their daily routine usually lead healthier, longer lives. Could LDN help prevent age-related disease deterioration and extend the human life span? I think it is quite possible.

It is also interesting to note that Tysabri, arguably the most effective of the conventional MS treatments available today, is now being used successfully to treat the inflammatory bowel condition, Crohn's disease. LDN, too, has been found to be an effective treatment for Crohn's. The April 2007 issue of the *Journal of Gastroenterology* published the results of a study carried out by Dr. Jill Smith and Dr. Ian Zagon at Penn State University. The study, titled "Low-dose naltrexone therapy improves active Crohn's disease," concludes that 67 percent of patients experienced complete remission and 89 percent experienced symptom improvement with LDN. The study concluded that LDN is safe and effective for patients with Crohn's disease, and that further studies on LDN for patients with Crohn's disease are warranted. (See http://www.ncbi.nlm.nih.gov/pubmed/17222320 and http://www.suite101.com/blog/daisyelaine/crohns_disease.)

Multiple sclerosis and Crohn's disease seem linked and Tysabri can effectively treat both. So apparently can LDN, but LDN costs less than a dollar a day and there is no risk of PML, as opposed to Tysabri costing over $130 a day and carrying a high risk of PML.

Immune-suppressing multiple sclerosis drug treatments, while somewhat effective, carry the risks of compromising the immune system, as well as possibly damaging the liver. People with MS may therefore be exposing themselves to significant dangers the longer they remain on these drugs. This was the case with the PML brain infections and resulting deaths that occurred from Tysabri. By compromising the body's immune system, the latent PML virus, present in everyone, was released.

The concept that you can treat a wide variety of debilitating autoimmune diseases with this generic drug that costs less than a dollar a day would be catastrophic to the for-profit US healthcare industry. Multiple sclerosis drugs alone represent an approximately $9 billion a year marketplace, not including the countless tests and doctors' visits involved. It is estimated that immune/inflammatory drug treatments in the US exceed over $68 billion a year, supporting approximately 375 drugs from 250 companies. (http://www.news-medical.net/news/20100105/Report-on-the-lucrative-immune inflammatory-disease-marketplace.aspx) These maintenance drugs are a continuing revenue stream. Yet, no one gets cured. Besides large drug companies, hospitals, doctors and medical technicians, autoimmune disease supports countless researchers, foundations and charitable organizations. LDN has the potential to turn this status quo on its head.

For multiple sclerosis, all it would take would be a relatively small clinical study to prove whether LDN is a superior first-line treatment for those newly diagnosed with the disease. Every day, approximately 200 people are diagnosed with MS in the United States. Take 200 of these people and give one hundred of them a standard beta-interferon treatment and the other one hundred, Low Dose Naltrexone. Conduct an MRI scan at the beginning of a two-year study and an MRI scan at the end, and measure plaque formation in the brain and spinal cord. All LDN needs is to be equal to 40 percent, or more effective than 40 percent, in slowing disease progression, and it becomes the preferable treatment in terms of administration, cost and toxicity. If LDN were shown to be more effective than beta-interferon treatment, it would validate the tens of thousands of user reports that LDN either completely halts disease progression or is 80 percent effective at slowing disease progression.

The lucrative US $9 billion multiple sclerosis drug marketplace would soon collapse.

Despite several large user surveys that consistently demonstrate that LDN is 80-85 percent effective in preventing MS, there has been a strong reluctance from the medical establishment to investigate conventional drug exacerbations. (http://www.ldners.org/surveys.htm) Even the National Multiple Sclerosis Society (NMSS) is highly resistant to supporting any meaningful LDN research. To date, NMSS has only directed $40,000 for a small study conducted on mice by Ian Zagon, PhD to determine whether LDN is safe. In that study done at Penn State, not only did no mice die, but those injected with the MS-like disease saw no progression while taking LDN. And those already taking LDN never came down with the MS-like disease. (http://autoimmunedisease.suite101.com/article.cfm/low_dose_naltrexone_in_experimental_model_of_ms) Despite these published results, the NMSS maintains the position that "further studies are needed to determine if LDN is safe for people with MS." NMSS has turned down all further LDN research study grant proposals from Penn State without comment.

It is estimated that well over 10,000 people worldwide currently take LDN for MS, and no one has died or reported life-threatening side effects. People who take LDN rarely stop taking it. Unfortunately, the four major multiple sclerosis drug manufacturers are major contributors to NMSS. One only needs to pick up a copy of the monthly edition of *MS Momentum* and see the full-page advertisements to understand their power and influence.

Every day 200 people walk into neurologists' offices and are given the devastating, life-changing news that they have MS. And every day 200 people do not hear about LDN. Instead, they are encouraged to take a drug treatment that is only 30-40 percent effective in slowing disease progression, requires weekly if not daily injections, carries unpleasant and often very toxic side effects, and costs over $2,500 a month, not including required tests and doctors' visits. They never hear about a non-toxic drug that may halt the disease in its tracks. It costs less than a dollar a day, is a nightly pill and makes you feel better. They will only hear about LDN if they aggressively search out alternative treatments for multiple sclerosis, or if they hear about LDN from a concerned friend. Most likely, they will only learn about LDN after their disease has progressed, after they have already experienced permanent damage to their myelin, and after they've lost their ability to walk. In other words, after the other drugs have failed. They will not hear about LDN from their neurologist. No neurologist will suggest taking LDN first because no pharmaceutical sales rep visits their office with free samples. There are no all-expenses-paid LDN conferences at golf resorts. No fancy dinners. No consulting fees.

What is going on is a modern medical tragedy. This is why I have joined well-known UK LDN advocate, Linda Elsegood, and several others to start www.LDNaware.org.

The mission of LDNaware.org is to raise public awareness of LDN. Our slogan is: "The more people who know about LDN, the more people will benefit from LDN." While a clinical trial proving the efficacy of LDN would indeed be valuable, it is unlikely that it will overcome the many obstacles the healthcare status quo will intentionally, and unintentionally, put in its path. The greatest resistance to LDN will always be found in the US, where a for-profit healthcare system prevents many lower-cost, or generic, treatments from being explored. In other countries, such as the UK, Germany, France, Australia, Canada and Japan, where health insurance does not distort market supply and demand forces, LDN is already gaining fast acceptance. People and governments simply cannot afford multiple sclerosis and other autoimmune therapies that cost in excess of $40,000-$50,000 per person, per year. In the UK, many MS-related organizations and charities have already embraced LDN, while their counterparts in the US have not. If the NMSS were to seriously consider supporting LDN research, they would risk angering their four drug company sponsors, and accordingly, their careers and lucrative salaries. (Joyce Nelson, CEO of NMSS, makes a $475,000-a-year salary. Source: NMSS.)

As a grassroots movement, LDNaware.org is a means of organizing the world community to effect change across many countries and cultures without the interference of for-profit interests.

LDN has changed my life. My MS-related symptoms have improved, and my disease does not seem to be progressing. However, I still walk with a cane or walker and require use of a wheelchair or scooter. I did not learn about LDN soon enough, so I have permanent damage to my cervical spine. It does not have to be this way for others, if they learn about LDN when their disease is first diagnosed. I envision the day when a neurologist will sit down with a terrified, newly diagnosed MS patient, and will recommend LDN as a first treatment, before the costly, toxic, injected drugs. The phrase as related to the common interpretation of the Hippocratic Oath, "First Do No Harm," would seem to apply to LDN.

I continue to tell everyone I know about LDN. My wife now takes LDN for her mild Crohn's disease that is now in remission. My 83-year-old father takes LDN for a Parkinson's-like disease that has now not progressed any further. His neurologist just shakes her head and keeps renewing the prescription. She has even started prescribing LDN for her MS patients who request it. They keep reporting positive results. My mother takes LDN for depression and has since stopped her Zoloft. The increased endorphins resulting from a nightly LDN pill make her just "feel better." Could LDN be a preferable treatment to the multi-billion-dollar antidepressant drug marketplace? I certainly think it is worth trying LDN first.

In business, a cash cow is "a product or a business unit that generates unusually high profit margins: so high that it is responsible for a large amount of a company's operating profit. This profit far exceeds the amount necessary to maintain the cash cow business, and the excess is used by the business for other purposes." (http://en.wikipedia.org/wiki/Cash_cow)

Every company wants a cash cow to milk. Multiple sclerosis and other autoimmune disease patients are the cash cows of pharmaceutical companies, specialists, hospitals and testing facilities. As long as these patients have good health insurance, they will be fed a never-ending supply of expensive drugs that require expensive visits to doctors who, in turn, prescribe more expensive tests. It is a never-ending cycle in which the patient never gets any better, but only "manages" his or her condition while waiting for the next drug to arrive. Perhaps it will be a drug that no longer requires painful injections, perhaps it will not harm your liver, or perhaps it will not make you feel sick after taking it. One thing is certain: If a pharmaceutical company makes it, you will have to take it forever, and it will cost a fortune.

Autoimmune disease treatment is a multi-billion-dollar marketplace that is only getting bigger. Better medical diagnostic equipment identifies MS earlier than ever before, and drug company-sponsored doctors recommend DMDs (disease-modifying drugs) as soon as possible.

Drug companies battle to show which drug is more effective with slick marketing of confusing clinical trial data to participants whose disease is characterized as "relapsing and remitting"—disease that comes and goes. The FDA is pressured by patients, doctors and drug companies to approve something for MS patients, even though, in clinical trials, all first-line MS drug treatments have been found to be really no more than 15 percent as effective as a placebo. The armies of attractive drug salespeople swarm doctors' offices bearing food and trinkets with sales targets of increasing prescription volumes. Paid celebrities make TV and conference appearances. Database marketing professionals collect user data, do telemarketing and direct mail, conduct customer satisfaction surveys and entertain their favored doctors, i.e., the ones who prescribe their drug the most. The NMSS holds endless walk- and bike-athons across the country to raise money for research, and most of that money goes to fund studies on drugs that are manufactured by pharmaceutical companies.

As I stated earlier, at the same time, the NMSS and its chapters pay their top executives lucrative salaries. Joyce Nelson, the CEO of NMSS, makes almost $500,000 a year, with many other top executives earning well over $250,000. Multiple sclerosis is a business and autoimmune disease is an industry.

Once acquired, an MS patient is worth between $30,000 and $50,000 a year for a pharmaceutical company, $2 million over a lifetime—a cash cow to be carefully milked until they can develop a new, improved and more expensive MS drug.

While I still have MS, I am no longer a cash cow. I take LDN. The more people who know about LDN, the more people benefit from LDN. Spread the word.

Malcolm's story is a very powerful "cautionary tale," of what happens when a patient follows the standard of care, when there are other treatments out there that might work better. Malcolm was quite lucky, in that his MS and the toxic, doctor-prescribed drugs he was taking didn't kill him—or further incapacitate him—before he found LDN. Now, thanks to Malcolm's tireless work, more people will hopefully discover LDN sooner than ever before. For more information on Malcolm's organization and his work, visit http://www.LDNaware.org.

I hope you have found the personal stories about each of these treatments to be as moving as I have. In most cases, I have found them motivational, too.

Their common message is: "There has to be a solution." I will elaborate further on this in the Afterword.

Listen to Your Gut!

I've learned so much from my experiences over the past twenty years, beginning with the fifteen years of being primary caretaker for my husband Tim, up to now, with the writing of this book. In addition to learning patience, which was not my strongest suit before Tim got sick, I learned about some stunning treatments that extended his life by at least twelve years. And, from working on this book—and especially from hearing the stories in it—I've learned that Mom was right. Whenever I had a seemingly unsolvable problem growing up, and while Tim was sick, too, my mom would repeat the mantra of one of my high school teachers, Dr. Christina Staël, and say, "There has to be a solution."

As I shared in the introduction to this book, my mom often told me the story of how in 1928 Dr. Charles Mayo—yes, *the* Charles Mayo—told my grandfather that my Grandma Julia's colon cancer was so far advanced that she had only six months to live. My mom was 11 years old—far too young to be left without a mother.

My grandfather's response (and I'm paraphrasing here, because "Papa Turitz" never swore) was a variation of "Like hell she does!" He then consulted his beloved "bible," *The Jewish Daily Forward*. At the time, a Dr. Chleminitsky was writing a regular column from Vienna, reporting on medical treatments outside the US that showed promise for treating all sorts of diseases. It was decided that one particular treatment, in Frankfurt-am-Main, Germany, was the most promising for my grandmother: radiation, combined with oxygen and carbon dioxide, then considered experimental in the United States.

So, in 1928, Grandma Julia, accompanied by one of her sons who knew German, made the trip to Germany. Long story short, Grandma Julia lived another eleven years—long enough to see my mom grow from an 11-year-old child to a graduate student at Columbia University. This experience fostered my mom's belief that "There has to be a solution."

Further, my mom believed that solution might be one your doctor doesn't know about. So, writing a book about lifesaving solutions to medical problems that doctors don't know about—and frankly, often don't want to know about—was in my DNA from a young age.

I feel honored that so many wonderful people were eager to have their inspiring stories included in my book. The fact that doctors, patient advocates and other experts joined together here makes this book so much more compelling, and special, for me. Now that you have read their stories, I hope you agree with me that, in most cases, "There has to be a solution." I also hope that you will not give up until you find the solution that is right for you. It really is possible for you to find treatments like these for your individual situation, and for the personal health situations of your friends and relatives.

I hope you will share my book and the wonderful stories in it with everyone you know who might be helped by the particular treatments described here. I hope you will also realize that these are not the only treatments out there that can help you and your loved ones. There are many others. It's just that your doctor probably won't tell you about them. In fact, chances are, he or she may not even know about them.

Another point of this book is that most doctors' interpretation of the words "patient empowerment" is just plain wrong. Most doctors view patient empowerment this way: They give you three (or four, or even five) options and together, you choose one of them. As I hope you've learned from this book, true empowerment often requires you to go that extra mile (or several miles) and do your own research. Go online. Talk to people. Then go back to your doctor with the treatments you have found, and together, choose the one that's right for you. If your doctor gets upset with you for believing that you are entitled to be a true partner in your own health care, find another doctor. (Or, as I am fond of quoting my doctor/dad as saying, "If your doctor tells you he knows all the answers, run like hell!" And unlike Papa Turitz, my dad did swear. I am quoting him verbatim!)

The standard of care is just that: the standard of care as practiced by most doctors in a particular area of specialization. But the medical establishment's standard of care should not necessarily be your personal standard of care. I want people to know that they can often, but not always, find answers that are better than their doctors' answers. I don't want you to ignore the good answers your doctor has. For instance, if we had not opted to have Tim's brain tumor surgically removed, he would have died in 1990, instead of 2005. There would have been nothing I could have done to help keep him alive for those fifteen additional years. We followed the doctors' advice when it made sense.

But I am asking you to filter your doctors' information, especially when the treatments they're recommending, or even insisting upon, are not working. Step outside the box and have the courage to start doing your own research. Let's be clear: It does take courage. And it certainly isn't easy. But it is easier than it once was. In the days when Jim Abrahams started looking for answers, he had to go to a physical library. We're all luckier today. We can research online; we can go into chat groups and forums. And here is something I haven't mentioned before: There are now lots of excellent professional consultants out there, who can help you by doing some very creative medical research. (I have listed two of these researchers in the Appendix.)

When you bring the results of your research to your doctor, don't be surprised if he or she scoffs at you. Remember what Dr. Berkson wrote in Chapter 4: Doctors are trained, not educated. Also remember the warnings of several of the patient advocates in this book, who warned against waiting too long to find treatments that work. Malcolm West told you that he is sure he would be less disabled today if he'd tried LDN when he first learned about it, rather than listening to his doctors and taking the medications they prescribed. Mary Bradley said the same thing. Additionally, every parent who wrote here about the Ketogenic Diet feels that his or her child would be much better off today if they had tried the diet earlier, before their children suffered from the exacerbations of their diseases and the side effects of the toxic drugs. Yet, their doctors all discouraged them from trying LDN and the Ketogenic Diet. Both Jean McCawley and Emma Williams even described how their children's doctors mocked them.

So, in this world of Internet research, know that the computer is your best friend. Start using it to do research now, before your medical condition, or that of a loved one, becomes desperate. Even my 93-year-old mother was once overheard saying, "God Bless Google."

If I had to put my advice into three simple words, they would be: Follow Your Gut. Only you can know if your doctor's way is not working. Start looking sooner, rather than later, before your disease progresses, before the toxic drugs you are taking cause side effects that become permanent.

And please take some time to review the postings on my website, www.HonestMedicine.com. I wrote there about Silverlon, intravenous alpha lipoic acid, the Ketogenic Diet and Low Dose Naltrexone long before I started to write this book. As I learn about other treatments and become convinced that they are as lifesaving, I will be writing about them as well.

So, please stay tuned. And please—once again—follow your gut. And when your gut tells you it is time to step out of the box, do it. To quote my Tim, your "tummy" will tell you when the time is right.

Thanks and Acknowledgments

I would like to thank those who have contributed chapters to this book: Jim Abrahams, Dr. Burt Berkson, Mary Jo Bean, Paul Marez, Millicent Kelly, Beth Zupec-Kania, Emma Williams, Jean McCawley, Dr. David Gluck, Linda Elsegood, Mary Boyle Bradley and Malcolm West. I would also like to thank Dr. Bernard Bihari, who was very ill at the time of the writing of this book. He died on May 16, 2010. Dr. Bihari's wife, Jackie Young, has been very helpful to me in the writing of this book. I want to thank her.

I'd also like to thank Margaret Schooling, Susan Popple and Daisy Zoll, who transcribed several of the LDN advocates' interviews that originally aired on Mary Boyle Bradley's Internet radio program. I used their transcriptions in my free e-book, *The Faces of Low Dose Naltrexone*, and adapted them for two of the LDN advocates' chapters in this book.

I'd also like to thank my parents. Growing up in their home made me a natural for writing *Honest Medicine*, since my parents both gave me a respect for nonconventional treatments and a skepticism concerning the medical establishment, a winning combination.

A big thanks to my mom, Sonya Schopick, whose openness to patient-evidence-based treatments stems from the fact that her own mother, my Grandma Julia, went to Germany in the late 1920s to try then-experimental radiation treatments, not yet available in the US. Thanks to these treatments, my grandmother lived eleven extra years, outliving her doctor by a few months. (You may read my grandmother's story here: http://www.honestmedicine.com/2006/08/another_inspira.html.) My mom, who is now 93 years old, has been one of my main supporters, urging me to get the word out about other patient-evidence-based treatments that could save lives today, just like the then-experimental radiation that extended her own mother's life in the 1920s.

And thanks to my dad, Dr. Louis Schopick, an MD who died over thirty years ago. He told me, even then, to be very wary of the medical establishment, that doctors don't know all the answers—not by a long shot. As I quoted him in the Afterword: "If a doctor tells you he knows all the answers, run like hell!"

You may read about my Dad, and his lack of love for the medical profession here: http://www.honestmedicine.com/2006/08/medicine_in_the.html.

I'll never forget how my brother Phil, my sister-in-law Carol, and my nephew and niece, Joe and Zara, were such wonderful supports to me while Tim was sick. They have been there for me ever since. Their sensitivity and love mean more to me than I can ever express to them. I'd also like to thank my sister, Fran, who called me faithfully whenever Tim was in the hospital. Her calls meant so much to me. And thanks, too, to my brothers, Daniel and David: Daniel for giving me legal advice over the years; and David, a doctor, for being open to holistic treatments, like those I feature in this book.

And there are some dear friends I'd like to thank:

Virginia McCullough, for being my friend and compatriot for so many years, and for spending hours brainstorming with me to figure out the best way to change the medical system. We soon decided that, while changing the system itself might be impossible, changing people's perceptions of it was possible. (Virginia is the co-author of several books about the medical system and so-called "anecdotal" treatments, including *The Oxygen Revolution: Hyperbaric Oxygen Therapy*, with Paul Harch, MD: http://www.amazon.com/Oxygen-Revolution-Hyperbaric-Groundbreaking-Disabilities/dp/1578262372/.) I shall always treasure her friendship.

A big thanks also goes to Karen Dean, who began as my editor at *Alternative and Complementary Therapies*, a publication for holistic medical professionals. In this capacity, she encouraged me to write some controversial articles that probably would never have been published had she not been editor. She and I have since become very good friends. Our long phone conversations, short visits and her salient bon mots always make me smile—especially her recent assessment (stated with near-awe) that, because of my pharmaceutical industry exposés on HonestMedicine.com, every pharmaceutical company probably has a dossier with my name on it! A compliment, indeed.

Thanks, too, to Leticia Thomas, who was more influential to me than even she knows. Leticia was the editor of *SEARCH*, the National Brain Tumor Foundation's newsletter, when I approached the publication about writing my article about how Silverlon healed Tim's non-healing skin. Leticia was instantly fascinated and supportive. I am sure it was because of Leticia's enthusiasm that our story appeared on the front page of the newsletter. Because of this, and because of what happened after my article appeared, which you learned about in Chapter 3, I was compelled to look for other treatments that doctors call "anecdotal," treatments that are, in fact, examples of patient-evidence-based medicine.

Thanks to my good friend, patient advocate Mary Shomon, whose books and websites about thyroid disease are an inspiration to me. For a list of her books on Amazon, go here: http://www.amazon.com/s/ref=nb_sb_noss?url=search-alias%3Dstripbooks&field-keywords=mary+shomon&x=0&y=0. Her websites are http://thyroid.about.com/ and http://www.thyroid-info.com/. Mary has a huge patient following. It is her inspiration that helped me know that a layperson/health writer can make one heck of a difference in this world. It is also Mary and her "let no grass grow under your feet" attitude that literally forced me to start my own website. While we were talking on the phone one day, Mary, growing tired of my almost constant talk of "I've got to start a website," took it upon herself to create one for me—that very day, while we were talking on the phone!

She emailed me the link, and HonestMedicine.com was off and running. I admire Mary more than I can say, and am happy to be able to call her my friend.

Thanks to radio talk show host and patient advocate, Kris Costello, who has not only encouraged me to write this book, but has nudged me along by threatening to post it on the Internet long before I thought it was "ready for prime time." You have no idea how her loving threats pushed me to get the book finished to my satisfaction. After my Mom, I think that Kris is my biggest fan. I am very grateful for her friendship and support. (See Kris's article, "My Hero: Julia Schopick," at http://www.wellnesstalkradio.com/hero-julia-shopick-honest-medicine/.)

Thanks to Chuck Poch, my computer guru. Without him, this book never would have been written, because every time my computer or Internet service went down, Chuck was there, performing his magic.

And thanks to Beth Barany, who, as my editor, added shape to a huge amount of information. Her enthusiasm for, and belief in, this book remained steadfast throughout a process that was sometimes rocky. She is a trusted friend and critic—a priceless combination.

A very special thanks to Dr. Carlos Reynes, who introduced me to Silverlon. And thanks also to Dr. Bart Flick, Silverlon's inventor. Dr. Reynes is now my personal physician, and Dr. Flick and I still keep in touch. I consider him to be a very good friend to this day. (You read about them both in Chapters 2 and 3.)

There are several other people I'd like to thank, including Jeanne Wallace, PhD, and her co-worker, Michelle Gerencser. I credit their nutritional advice with giving Tim a great many additional years of life. Jeanne and Michelle have both been wonderful friends, supportive of me and my work. And thanks, too, to my good friend, nutritionist Liz Lipski, PhD, and her former assistant Aubrey Mast.

Liz and I have worked together and been friends for over twenty years. I will always be grateful for her many kindnesses.

And of course, Tim's and my dear friend, Keith Peterson, to whom Tim—although he had no formal will—left his substantial book collection. I include Keith here because, although he has absolutely no interest in healthcare, he has read almost every word I've written, and has provided me with some very helpful suggestions. And thanks to Keith for the author photo on the back of this book.

There are also many other friends who have been supportive, including Beth Ryza and Harry Steckman, Rose Nelson, Ann McCabe, Victoria Manning, Victoria Pratt, Michael James Moore, Bianca Zola, Mick Aber, Celia Daniels, Ruth and Jerry Moyar, David Dalton, Chuck Powers, Daphne White, Tracey Cymbal, Cathy Lewis, Shelvia Tinsley, Ginny Lazzara and Kathy Bezinovich.

Thanks, too, to those who have spread the word about my work and about my site, www.HonestMedicine.com, including Mary Jo Bean. Mary Jo has been a great help to me by reaching out to several of Dr. Berkson's patients, and telling them about this book. In addition, I'd like to thank each and every one of the LDN patient advocates, including those who have not contributed chapters. They, too, have been very supportive of this book. Unfortunately, there are far too many to name all of them here.

Thanks, too, to the generous professionals who have written the testimonials at the beginning of this book and on the cover: Drs. Julian Whitaker, Ronald Hoffman, Jeffrey Dach, David Brownstein and Jacob Teitelbaum. Also, Virginia McCullough, Mary Shomon, Kris Costello and Jackie Young.

And special thanks, too, to my very good friend Mark, who showed me that there is not only one man in the world for each woman. I know it's trite to say this, but, in the words of Debbie Boone: Mark, you light up my life!

But most of all, I want to thank Tim. With him, I found the kind of love it took to inspire me to try so hard to find treatments that might extend his life, no matter how non-standard-of-care those treatments might be. It was Tim who trusted me one hundred percent when no one before him ever had, and who talked me up, whenever people remarked how well he was doing—at least for the first eleven years after his original diagnosis. "She's a doctor's daughter," he'd tell them. "She knows everything." (While I was a doctor's daughter, I think his assessment was a bit over the top!)

Ironically, I first learned about each of the treatments contained in this book while researching treatments for Tim. Even though I didn't use every one of these treatments for him, Tim really is the glue that holds these pages together.

Appendix

This Appendix contains information that I promised within the text of this book, along with other information I think is important for you to have. In some cases, I include entire articles. But more often, the information is in the form of hyperlinks to websites or to PDF files where you can go to read more about a particular topic. My computer contains a huge amount of information, which I amassed both prior to and during the writing of this book. So, if you have any questions, or would like to know more about any relevant topic covered in this book that isn't here, please write to me at Julia@HonestMedicine.com. The fact that I didn't include a particular study, article or other piece of information here does not mean that I don't have it in my files. If I do have it, I'll be happy to share it with you.

OUTLINE FOR THE CONTENTS OF THIS APPENDIX

SECTION 1: WELCOME TO THE WORLD OF LOW-COST, INNOVATIVE TREATMENTS THAT WORK

1. Selected Articles by and about Julia Schopick, Published in Professional Publications

2. Medical Researchers

3. Nutritionists

4. General Health Websites

SECTION 2: INTRAVENOUS ALPHA LIPOIC ACID

1. Dr. Burt Berkson's Nutritional Program

2. Dr. Burt Berkson's List of Prescribed Supplements

3. Dr. Berkson's Books

4. Dr. Berkson's Hepatitis and Cancer Studies, and Interviews

5. Dr. Berkson's Videos and Audios

6. Dr. Berkson's Favorite Quote (from *The Lancet*)

7. "Pharmaceutical News by Press Release? (OR: Low Dose Naltrexone Study Doesn't Make the News)," an article from HonestMedicine.com

SECTION 3: THE KETOGENIC DIET

1. Ketogenic Diet History

2. Historical Case Studies/Ketogenic Diet Studies—1920s to 1990s

3. About The Charlie Foundation

4. Link to The Consensus Statement

5. Link to the *Mayo Clinic Bulletin*, 1921

6. Resources from Emma Williams and Matthew's Friends

7. Article on Brain Tumors and the Ketogenic Diet

8. Milly Kelly: A Brief Summary of the Hospital Routine—Full Text

9. The Stevens Johnson Syndrome Foundation

10. A Ketogenic Diet Support Group

11. Links to Ketogenic Diet Pages on Facebook

12. ACTH Versus the Ketogenic Diet: Comparative Efficacy

13. Article by Diana Pillas: "The Implementation and Maintenance of the Ketogenic Diet in Children"

SECTION 4: LDN

1. Five Main LDN Websites that Link to Other Sites

2. Online LDN Forums

3. LDN Studies

4. Compounding Pharmacies

5. Doctors who Prescribe LDN

6. Ian Zagon, PhD: Primary LDN Researcher

7. Media Coverage of Dr. Bihari

8. Dr. Bihari's Proposal to the Irish Government to do a Trial on LDN for MS—Full Text

9. LDN Fact Sheets (to Educate Your Doctor About LDN)

10. HonestMedicine.com's Articles about LDN

~

SECTION 1: WELCOME TO THE WORLD OF LOW-COST, INNOVATIVE TREATMENTS THAT WORK

1. Selected Articles by and about Julia Schopick, Published in Professional Publications

For a few years before Tim was diagnosed with a brain tumor, I had been an intermittent contributor to the AMA publication, *American Medical News*. Since I was a public relations consultant whose clients included physicians, my columns instructed physicians on how to market their practices.

Soon after Tim got sick, it became clear to me that all the marketing know-how in the world wouldn't help doctors build their practices if they didn't know how to communicate with patients. And, every day, I was learning anew about doctors' severe deficiencies in this area. So, I approached my editor at *AMA News* about writing articles to educate doctors about how to communicate effectively with patients. She agreed.

Below is a list of the series of articles I wrote. In one case, the column is no longer online. There, I give just the title. In cases where the articles or columns are online, and are only accessible with a subscription to the publication, I am providing the link. If you do not have a subscription, and want to read a particular article, please contact me at Julia@HonestMedicine.com, and I'll be glad to send you a copy of the article.

- "Four Basic Rules Help Doctors Avoid Alienating Patients," December 23/30, 1991

- "Hippocrates was right: Treat people, not their disease," June 26, 2000. http://www.ama-assn.org/amednews/2000/06/26/hlca0626.htm

- "Empowered patients may have something to teach," September 25, 2000. http://www.ama-assn.org/amednews/2000/09/25/hlca0925.htm

- "Doctors can deliver hope as well as facts of prognosis," March 12, 2001. http://198.178.213.111/amednews/2001/03/12/hlca0312.htm

- A review in the *British Medical Journal* of an anthology in which one of my *AMA News* articles was featured. (The review focuses specifically on my article.) http://careers.bmj.com/careers/advice/view-article.html?id=558

I also wrote several articles that were published in *Alternative and Complementary Therapies* magazine, a professional publication for holistic health practitioners. Some of these articles are about treatments (e.g., hyperbaric oxygen therapy) that, like the ones I profile in this book, are inexpensive alternatives to treatments for conditions conventional medicine does not treat very effectively.

- "Drug-Nutrient Interactions: Leo Galland, MD, Discusses His New Database," April 2005.

  Since many patients now take a combination of drugs and nutritional supplements, this drug-nutrient database should be used by all doctors, conventional and alternative alike.

  http://honestmedicine.typepad.com/GallandFINAL.pdf

- "Exploring Stem Cell Therapy Potentials: A Q&A with Anthony G. Payne, PhD," June 2005.

  A serious look at using adult stem cells for neurological disorders.

  http://honestmedicine.typepad.com/StemCells-FINAL-June-21-05.pdf

- "Could Alternative Medicine Have Saved Terri Schiavo?" June 2005.

  An exploration of whether hyperbaric oxygen therapy could have brought Terri Schiavo out of her coma.

  http://honestmedicine.typepad.com/Schiavo-FINAL.pdf

2. Medical Researchers

Throughout this book, I recommend that people research solutions to their health problems, especially in cases where they are not happy with the solutions their doctors are recommending. But, the truth is that not all of us have the know-how and wherewithal to do this research by ourselves. For this reason, I am including the names of two researchers who have a great deal of credibility and experience. There are many others. These are the two I have dealt with personally.

a. Janice Guthrie—The Health Resource

http://www.thehealthresource.com/

Not long after Tim was diagnosed with a brain tumor, I realized that, if he was to have a long survival, I needed to go beyond the advice our doctors were providing. One day, while reading an article in a major women's magazine, I found Jan Guthrie. Her personal story of being a long-time cancer survivor was inspiring. And the fact that, for a very reasonable price, she provided me with personalized research, totally tailored to Tim's individual health situation, was reassuring. I hired Jan several times over the years, when a new health crisis came up (e.g., intractable seizures, shunt failure, etc.) and have recommended her services to many other people. (Jan researches diseases and conditions other than cancer, too.)

b. Ralph Moss, PhD. Cancer Decisions

http://www.cancerdecisions.com/

Dr. Moss is well known in the alternative cancer community as the author of several books that are critical of conventional cancer treatments, i.e., "the Cancer Industry." Dr. Moss also supplies reports to patients on various kinds of cancer; his emphasis is on natural solutions, as opposed to chemotherapy and radiation. His reports are not individualized, the way Jan Guthrie's are. But because of his long history of being involved in reporting on cancer treatments, I usually advise cancer patients to purchase his excellent reports, along with Jan Guthrie's.

3. Nutritionists

For the first several years Tim got sick, we did not look to nutrition as part of the solution, beyond, of course, our doctors' advice to "eat a healthy diet." Then my friend Bianca Zola told me she had read about a nutritionist, Jeanne Wallace, PhD, whose area of specialization was cancer, with a particular emphasis on brain tumors. I called Jeanne. Along with Jan Guthrie, I credit her with extending Tim's life by many years.

    a. Jeanne Wallace, PhD

       http://nutritional-solutions.net/

       You may find the testimonial I wrote about Jeanne on her website.

    b. Michelle Gerencser

       http://www.lymphomanutrition.com/Home.html

       Michelle is Jeanne's assistant. Over the years, she has become the "go-to" nutritionist for all things related to lymphomas. I highly recommend her, as well.

    c. Elizabeth Lipski, PhD

       http://www.innovativehealing.com/

       Dr. Lipski was my first public relations client. She is an excellent all-round nutritionist, and I always refer people to her who have digestive problems. Liz is the author of *Digestive Wellness*, one of the most respected books on this topic. (Digestion is extremely important because many illnesses result from problems that start in the digestive tract.) My interview with Liz is at http://www.honestmedicine.com/2006/09/1_interview_wit.html.

4. General Health Websites

    a. Annie Appleseed Project: An excellent website for patients with cancer. Ann Fonfa, the founder, is herself a many-year survivor of breast cancer. She is an inspiration.

       http://www.annieappleseedproject.org/

b. Innovative Healing: Nutritionist Liz Lipski, PhD's website. This site has lots of information about nutritional solutions for many health problems. Contains articles, video clips and more.

http://www.innovativehealing.com/

c. Nutritional Solutions: Jeanne Wallace, PhD's website. This site also contains a great deal of information, with a slant toward nutritional treatments for people with cancer who are going through traditional treatment protocols (i.e., surgery, chemotherapy, radiation). Pay special attention to Jeanne's excellent articles.

http://nutritional-solutions.net/

d. Cancer Decisions: Ralph Moss, PhD's website. This site contains a huge amount of information. Dr. Moss, the author of many books about the downside of conventional cancer treatments, has a wonderful weekly newsletter. I highly recommend that you sign up for it.

http://www.cancerdecisions.com/

SECTION 2: INTRAVENOUS ALPHA LIPOIC ACID

1. Dr. Burt Berkson's Nutritional Program

This program is customized to each patient's individual needs. Always check with your practitioner for support.

Integrative Medical Center of New Mexico
Burton M. Berkson, MD, MS, PhD, President
575-524-3720

Simple Nutritional Programs

Fresh Green Vegetables—4-6 per day: Cabbage, broccoli, spinach, cauliflower, cilantro, greens

Fresh Whole Grains: Cooked oatmeal, rice, barley, corn, buckwheat, groats

Proteins: Whole eggs, roast chicken, fresh fish, beans, block cheeses, occasional red meat

Fats: Genuine butter, olive oil

Fluids: Water, tea, non-decaffeinated coffee, fresh vegetable juice

AVOID
Milk by the glass
White flour and white sugar
Diet foods
Restaurant deep-fried foods
Margarine
Tobacco
Salty foods
Alcohol (liver patients)

MUST HAVE
High fiber foods
Exercise
Bowel movement every day
Fun
Reduce stress

2. **Dr. Burt Berkson's List of Prescribed Supplements**

Any supplement and vitamin program is specially designed for each individual patient and must be reviewed with your doctor. The dosages and supplements are individualized for each patient. This list is a guideline only.

Integrative Medical Center of New Mexico
Burton M. Berkson, MD, MS, PhD, President
575-524-3720

Simple Nutritional Program/Supplements

All supplements and vitamins must NOT be exposed to heat. Store in a cool, dry place.

Multivitamin with minerals (no iron)
Vitamin C
Vitamin E
Elderberry/Zinc
Alpha lipoic acid
B-Complex
Selenium
Silymarin
IP6
Pantothenic Acid
Chromium Picolinate
L-Carnitine
Pancreatin
L-Glutamine
L-Arginine
Melatonin

NAC
CoQ10
ACUTE IMMUNITY (sinus/respiratory)
Beta Carotene
Bilberry
Lutein
Lycopene
Saw Palmetto
Pros-tech
Zinc Picolinate
Andro Dim
Cranberry
Pro Omega
Salmon Oil
Probiotic XS
Phytocort
Rebuild
Vitamin D
Horse Chestnut
Chondroitin Sulfate
Glucosamine Sulfate
MSM
Zyflamend
AHCC
Laktoferrin
NAC
Nattokinase
Artemisinin
Magnesium citrate Dim (Diindolylmethane)
Gingko Phytosome (Morningstar Minerals)
Psyllium
Boswellia
Curcumin

3. **Dr. Berkson's Books: (Available at fine bookstores everywhere)**

   a. *The Alpha Lipoic Acid Breakthrough: The Superb Antioxidant That May Slow Aging, Repair Liver Damage, and Reduce the Risk of Cancer, Heart Disease, and Diabetes*

   b. *Syndrome X: The Complete Nutritional Program to Prevent and Reverse Insulin Resistance*, co-author with Jack Challem and Melissa Diane Smith

   c. *User's Guide to the B-Complex Vitamins*, co-author, with Arthur J. Berkson

4. **Dr. Berkson's Hepatitis and Cancer Studies and Interviews**

a. Dr. Berkson's paper, co-authored with F. C. Bartter, J. Gallelli and P. Hiranaka, "Thioctic Acid in the Treatment of Poisoning with Alpha-Amanitin." Presented at the International Amanita Symposium, Heidelberg, Germany, November 1-3, 1978.

http://honestmedicine.typepad.com/BERKSON-1980-amanitin.pdf

b. Dr. Berkson's first short note on treating liver disease. Published in the *New England Journal of Medicine.*

http://www.ncbi.nlm.nih.gov/pubmed/366411?ordinalpos=3&itool=EntrezSystem2.PEntrez.Pubmed.Pubmed_Results Panel.Pubmed_DefaultReportPanel.Pubmed_RVDocSum

c. Dr. Berkson's Cancer Papers

- "The Long-term Survival of a Patient With Pancreatic Cancer With Metastases to the Liver After Treatment With the Intravenous α-Lipoic Acid/Low-Dose Naltrexone Protocol." *Integr. Cancer Ther.* Vol. 5, No. 1, 83-89. (2006)

  http://www.ldn4cancer.com/files/Berkson_Pancreatic_paper.pdf; http://ict.sagepub.com/content/5/1/83.short

- "Revisiting the ALA/N (a-Lipoic Acid/Low-Dose Naltrexone) Protocol for People With Metastatic and Nonmetastatic Pancreatic Cancer: A Report of 3 New Cases." *Integr. Cancer Ther.* Vol. 8, No. 4, 416-22. (2009)

  http://www.magicwater.org/storage/Case%20study%20Pancreatic%20cancer%20ALA-LDN.pdf

d. "Lipoic Acid Breakthrough," An interview of Dr. Burt Berkson by Richard A. Passwater, PhD, *Whole Foods Magazine*, October 2005.

http://www.drpasswater.com/nutrition_library/Nov_05/Berkson_Lipoic_final.html

5. **Dr. Berkson's Videos and Audios**

   a. LDN 2008, Dr. Burt Berkson, "Best of, Parts 1-4." In the next four videos, Dr. Berkson speaks about intravenous alpha lipoic acid and LDN for a patient with pancreatic cancer. This video series comes from his speech at the 2008 LDN conference. As you will hear in the videos, according to Dr. Berkson, ALA is just as important as, or even more important than, LDN to his treatment protocol.

   Part 1: http://www.youtube.com/watch?v=WqRwXEnPYKk

   Part 2: http://www.youtube.com/watch?v=4bpRai9S03A

   Part 3: http://www.youtube.com/watch?v=BLoS_U85g0Y

   Part 4: http://www.youtube.com/watch?v=wxVUimTW6sQ

   b. Keynote speaker at a 2009 LDN conference:

   http://www.youtube.com/watch?v=WHyUfHqR4PA

   c. HonestMedicine.com's interview with Dr. Berkson: "Audio Interview: Burt Berkson, MD, MS, PhD, Talks With Honest Medicine About His Work With Alpha Lipoic Acid and Low Dose Naltrexone"

   http://www.honestmedicine.com/2009/02/audio-interview-burt-berkson-md-phd-talks-with-honest-medicine-about-his-work-with-alpha-lipoic-acid.html

   A link to the transcript of this interview is also available here.

6. **Dr. Burt Berkson's Favorite Quote (from *The Lancet*, the respected British medical publication)**

   "If everything has to be double-blinded, randomized, and evidence-based, where does that leave new ideas?"
   —*The Lancet*, Vol. 366, #9480, pages 95-176, July 9-15, 2005.

The quote was on the cover of Vol. 366, #9480, and refers to an editorial in this issue titled "Could Evidence Based Medicine Be a Danger to Progress? If everything has to be double-blinded, randomized, and evidence-based, where does that leave new ideas?"

7. **"Pharmaceutical News by Press Release? (OR: Low Dose Naltrexone Study Doesn't Make the News)" from Honest Medicine.com**

The study described in this HonestMedicine.com article is referred to by Dr. Berkson in Chapter 4. It describes a paper that a doctor presented at a meeting of the American Academy of Neurology in April 2008. This paper, which reported on a successful LDN trial in Italy, received no publicity. Instead, another MS drug trial that was reported on at the meeting received heavy coverage in the press. The difference: The drug trial that received the publicity was funded by a large pharmaceutical company while the LDN trial, of course, was not.

http://www.honestmedicine.com/2009/02/pharmanews.html

Section 3: The Ketogenic Diet

1. **Ketogenic Diet History**

   a. http://en.wikipedia.org/wiki/Ketogenic_diet

   b. For another article that gives a tremendous amount of information about the diet, historically and medically, go to State-of-the-Art Review Article: "The Ketogenic Diet: One Decade Later," by John M. Freeman, MD, Eric H. Kossoff, MD, Adam L. Hartman, MD. March 1, 2007, *PEDIATRICS* Vol. 119 No. 3 March 2007, pp. 535-543. (doi:10.1542/peds.2006-2447)

   http://pediatrics.aappublications.org/cgi/content/full/119/3/535

   c. Also: "High Fat and Seizure Free," *Johns Hopkins Magazine*, Electronic Edition, April 1995. An excellent article for historical information on the diet.

   http://www.jhu.edu/jhumag/495web/fat.html

   d. The following two articles are about Chester ("Chet") White, Jr., who was treated by Dr. Samuel Livingston at Johns Hopkins in the 1940s. Today, Mr. White is in his mid-60s, and is able to eat all foods without experiencing seizures. In fact, he calls himself a "carbohydrate junkie."

http://www.charliefoundation.org/ketokids/chets-story

http://www.epilepsy.com/epilepsy/keto_news_dec08

2. **Historical Case Studies/Ketogenic Diet Studies (Provided by Jim Abrahams)**

   a. 1920s through 1950s:

   http://honestmedicine.typepad.com/Ketogenic%20Diet%20Studies-Part%201-1920s%20to%201950s.pdf

   b. 1960s through 1990s:

   http://honestmedicine.typepad.com/Ketogenic%20Diet%20Studies-Part2-1960s-1990s.pdf

3. **About The Charlie Foundation**

   http://charliefoundation.org/

The Charlie Foundation was established in 1994 in order to raise awareness about the Ketogenic Diet as a treatment for childhood epilepsy. The modern success of the diet has led to new demands on the medical community. In order to meet these demands, The Charlie Foundation has expanded its priorities to include educational programs for dietitians and neurologists as well as support for clinicians and researchers working to perfect its administration and discover its mechanisms.

The Charlie Foundation has a wealth of information on its site: http://charliefoundation.org/

   a. Photos

   In addition to the FAQs, and listing of events (past and present), there are lots of photos on The Charlie Foundation website. My favorite is this photo of Jim, Nancy and Charlie, right after Charlie was cured with the Ketogenic Diet. Note Jim's expression of victory!

   http://charliefoundation.org/gallery/charlie-nancy-jim-people-magazine

b. Hospitals that Administer the Ketogenic Diet

This site also contains an amazingly valuable list of the hospitals in the US and abroad that have Ketogenic Diet programs.

http://charliefoundation.org/hospitals

c. "Dateline NBC" Videos on YouTube, The Charlie Foundation Channel

- "Dateline" video, Part 1

  http://www.youtube.com/watch?v=STPOEFfQdjw

- "Dateline" video, Part 2

  http://www.youtube.com/watch?v=VdP9JyYgasA

d. Videos on The Charlie Foundation Website

http://www.charliefoundation.org

Under the photo of Meryl Streep, there are several thumbnails. Click on each one for a different video. Among those whose videos are featured:

- Julie McCawley

- Emma Williams

- Charlie Abrahams

- Dr. Deborah Snyder

- Several segments from Jim's made-for-television movie, "First Do No Harm."

  At http://www.charliefoundation.org/medical_opinions, you will find videos of several doctors who use the Ketogenic Diet to treat children. Among them:

- Eileen PG Vining, MD, Johns Hopkins Hospital, Baltimore, MD

- Greg L. Holmes, MD, Dartmouth-Hitchcock Medical Center, Lebanon, NH

- J. Helen Cross, MD, PhD, Great Ormond Street Hospital/Institute of Child Health, London, UK

- Jong M. Rho, MD, Barrow Neurological Institute, Phoenix, AZ

- Elizabeth Thiele, MD, PhD, Massachusetts General Hospital, Boston, MA

- James W. Wheless, MD, Le Bonheur Children's Medical Center, Nashville, TN

- Christina Bergqvist, MD, Children's Hospital of Philadelphia, PA

- Eric Kossoff, MD, Johns Hopkins Hospital, Baltimore, MD

- Elaine Wirrell, MD, Mayo Clinic, Rochester, MN

- Ruth E. Williams, MD, Evelina Children's Hospital, London, UK

e. Low Carbohydrate Recipes

Low-Carb and Carb-Free Products

http://www.charliefoundation.org/content/low-carb-and-carb-free-products

Keto Recipes

http://charliefoundation.org/recipes

4. Link to The Consensus Statement

"SPECIAL REPORT: Optimal clinical management of children receiving the Ketogenic Diet: Recommendations of the International Ketogenic Diet Study Group," better known as The Consensus Statement. Published in *Epilepsia*, the premier publication for neurologists, this article advocates that the diet be made available as a treatment after two anti-epileptic medicines have been tried and have failed.

http://honestmedicine.typepad.com/consensus_statement.pdf

5. Link to the *Mayo Clinic Bulletin*, 1921

By Dr. R. M. Wilder, one of the pioneers of the Ketogenic Diet, this is one of the first studies ever published about the diet. Jim Abrahams provided me with this resource.

http://honestmedicine.typepad.com/MayoBulletin_1921.pdf

6. Resources from Emma Williams and Matthew's Friends

Matthew's Friends: http://site.matthewsfriends.org/

A registered charity in the United Kingdom, all information on the Matthew's Friends site is downloadable for families and health care professionals to be accessible to everyone. Matthew's Friends has a medical board whose aim is to empower parents to ask the right questions and give them confidence to stand up for their children and not feel guilty about such actions.

This site contains a wealth of information, including:

   a. Descriptions of the various variations of the diet, including the MCT Diet and the Modified Atkins Diet

   b. Medical papers:
      http://site.matthewsfriends.org/index.php?page=medical-papers

   c. A professional forum

   d. A patient/parent forum

   e. Videos on YouTube, such as:

      i. Emma Williams' speech at The Charlie Foundation April 2008—International Symposium on Diet Therapies in Phoenix, Arizona
         http://www.youtube.com/watch?v=T7DQOAeFFQo

      ii. Preparing yourself, your family, and your child for the Ketogenic Diet: A Parent
         http://www.epilepsy.com/epilepsy/keto_news_june07

      iii. Matthew's story: http://www.charliefoundation.org/keto kids/matthews-story

7. Article on Brain Tumors and the Ketogenic Diet

"Targeting energy metabolism in brain cancer: review and Hypothesis," *Nutrition & Metabolism* 2005, 2:30 doi: 10.1186 /1743-7075-2-30. Thomas N Seyfried and Purna Mukherjee.

This article is important because it shows that the Ketogenic Diet is now being used for other medical conditions, in addition to epilepsy.

http://www.nutritionandmetabolism.com/content/2/1/30

8. Milly Kelly: A Brief Summary of Hospital Routine

As you read in Milly Kelly's chapter (Chapter 8), the Ketogenic Diet must be administered carefully in order for the child to experience success. Either the child experiences the complete elimination of seizures, or if that is not possible, a reduction in their number.

For either of these results to happen, when the child is first put on the diet, he or she must be hospitalized and carefully monitored until ketosis is reached. (Ketosis is the state where the body thinks it is fasting, and uses fat rather than glucose for energy.)

To assure the greatest success with the diet, the dietitians and family need to start working together for several days, or even weeks, before the child is admitted to the hospital.

Milly Kelly was a dietitian at Johns Hopkins from 1948 to 1998. She prepared this description.

PRIOR TO ADMISSION
Once the child's hospital admission date has been set, the dietitian contacts the parents by phone, and gathers the information needed to devise each individual patient's diet. This information includes the child's birth date, age, height, weight, eating habits, food likes and dislikes, medicines, seizure types and food allergies. The dietitian then calculates the diet and makes at least twelve meal plans for each individual child.

ON THE DAY BEFORE ADMISSION
The patient and family attend classes in the outpatient pediatric seizure clinic with the dietitian. The purpose of the diet and the hospitalization routine are explained, and the family is given various handouts.

Among them: the twelve meal plans that have been prepared specifically for the family's child.

Fasting starts after the evening meal, bringing about the depletion of glucose, which then leads to ketosis.

ON DAY 1

The patient is admitted to the hospital. Fasting continues. During the fast, fluids are given in the form of zero-calorie decaffeinated beverages only. Acceptable fluids include water, sugar-free lemonade, decaffeinated tea, sugar-free/decaffeinated sodas. The amount of liquid each child receives during the fasting period, and continued during the diet, is based on the number of calories prescribed in their diet plan. Fluids must be divided throughout the day, not to exceed more than 120 to 150 ccs per serving. (Editor's note: 120 ccs is about 4 fluid oz.; 150 ccs is about 5 fluid oz.)

It is important not to give too many (or too few) fluids during the fasting or the diet phase. Too much fluid can wash out the ketones, thereby diminishing the ketogenic effects of the diet. Similarly, if the child doesn't get enough liquids, he or she may become too acidotic. Acidosis is an extreme and dangerous form of ketosis. This is why it is crucial that the diet be started in the hospital under medical supervision, and not at home. (Editor's note: Please read Milly's chapter, Chapter 8, for an excellent description of ketones and ketosis.)

DAY 2 AND THEREAFTER

Fasting continues until the child is in ketosis. Some children come into the hospital already in ketosis, because their parents have had them fasting at home. But most do not. So they usually need to fast for approximately twenty-hour to forty-eight hours in the hospital before the desired level of ketosis (4+ on the dipstick) is reached. Once this level is reached, the physician in charge will write an order to start feeding.

Food is introduced slowly. On the first day of the diet, one-third of the child's total daily calories are given in the form of a special preparation of "Ketogenic Eggnog," divided into three equal meals labeled #1, #2 and #3. On the second day, the child progresses to two-thirds of the total calories of Ketogenic Eggnog, again divided into three equal meals, labeled #4, #5 and #6. On the third day, they will get their first solid meal: Meal #7. From then on, they will be fed a solid diet, restricted to the number of calories that have been calibrated for that particular child.

Patients and family members attend daily scheduled classes with the dietitian, learning how to use the gram scale, and how to prepare and serve meals and fluids. In one of the classes, a nurse teaches parents about what to do during sick days—in other words, whether to keep feeding the child, if he or she isn't hungry, etc. In these classes, parents are able to ask questions and get answers from both dietitian and nurse, and to become acquainted with each other.

Once the child has had two to three full meals and medications have been adjusted, he or she is ready for discharge. Special eggnog calculated specifically for each child is prepared for the journey home. Follow-up appointments are made. Changes in the diet and in the ratios of calories, fats, proteins and carbohydrates will be made as needed.

9. The Stevens Johnson Syndrome Foundation

The Stevens Johnson Syndrome Foundation is Jean McCawley's organization. She set it up to disseminate information about this horrible condition that her daughter Julie contracted as a baby from taking her first anti-seizure medication, Phenobarbital.

http://www.sjsupport.org/

10. A Ketogenic Diet Support Group

Ciros Centrum: A website in German, created by Austrian parents, Veronica and Helmut Blum, whose child was cured by the Ketogenic Diet.

http://www.ciros-centrum.com/ihre_hilfe/so_helfen_sie_uns.htm

11. Links to Ketogenic Diet Pages on Facebook

a. Ketogenic Diet for Epilepsy Group:

http://www.facebook.com/#!/group.php?gid=2444070101&ref=ts

b. Ketogenic Diet:

There are other websites for the Ketogenic Diet on Facebook. Just search for the term in the search bar:

http://www.facebook.com/#!/pages/Ketogenic-Diet/275458737515?ref=ts

12. ACTH Versus the Ketogenic Diet: Comparative Efficacy

When I first began writing *Honest Medicine*, I planned to include a section titled "ACTH Versus the Ketogenic Diet" as the perfect example of the medical profession's penchant for using expensive, side-effect-laden treatments instead of treatments like the ones featured in this book.

The comparison was perfect: ACTH and the Ketogenic Diet are both effective for a condition called infantile spasms. However, ACTH is extremely costly: approximately $200,000 to $250,000 a month, or $480,000 to $720,000 for two to three months, the average length of time babies had to stay on it. ACTH also has terrible side effects. Still, until recently, doctors preferred it to the Ketogenic Diet. During the writing of this book, many insurance companies stopped covering the cost of ACTH, and the use of the Ketogenic Diet increased. However, many doctors now prescribe prednisone for this condition, instead of the Ketogenic Diet.

I believe it is still important to include this information here, so that you will see the kind of money insurance companies routinely pay, instead of covering these safer, less expensive treatments.

In April 2008, a study comparing the two treatments, conducted by Drs. Kossoff, Hedderick, Turner and Freeman, was published in *Epilepsia*, the primary journal for professionals who treat patients with epilepsy. The study compared both the efficacy and safety of the Ketogenic Diet with ACTH. The conclusion: "In this retrospective study, the Ketogenic Diet stopped spasms in nearly two-thirds of cases, and had fewer side effects and relapses than ACTH."

Abstracts on this study are here:

http://www.ncbi.nlm.nih.gov/pubmed/18410363

and here:

http://www3.interscience.wiley.com/journal/120120297/abstract?CRETRY=1&SRETRY=0

Additionally, an abstract was presented at the American Epilepsy Society meeting in December 2009, showing that all of the babies that they put on the ketogenic formula had significant improvement in seizure control: 100 percent.

http://www.aesnet.org/go/publications/aes-abstracts/abstract-search/?mode=display&sy=2009&sb=all&startrow=811&id=9658

13. **Article by Diana Pillas: "The Implementation and Mainte-nance of the Ketogenic Diet in Children," in the *Journal of Neuroscience Nursing*, October 1, 1999**

Diana Pillas was a nurse at Johns Hopkins when Milly Kelly was there, and for several years thereafter. This article by Diana Pillas is the most complete description of the Ketogenic Diet that I have read.

http://www.allbusiness.com/health-care-social-assistance/nursing-residential/357056-1.html

SECTION 4: LDN

There is no question that Low Dose Naltrexone probably has more patient and physician sites—websites, forums, blogs, etc.—devoted to it than the other treatments featured in this book. In order to avoid missing some of them, instead of trying to list them all, I will link to the primary sites, which themselves contain links to the others.

1. **Five Main LDN Websites that Link to Other Sites**

    a. http://LDNaware.org/

    This site has links to websites and blogs all around the world, listed by country, and is continually adding more sites and resources as they become known. So, if you find that your site is not included there, please contact LDNaware.org.

    b. http://www.LDNers.org/

    SammyJo Wilkinson's site. See especially the resource page: http://www.ldners.org/resources.htm, where there are links to the LDN forums.

    c. http://LDNinfo.org/

    (Also http://lowdosenaltrexone.org/, which is the same site.) This site also has links to all the media (videos and audios) from the LDN conferences, as well as to the studies worldwide.

    d. http://www.LDNResearchTrust.org/

    Linda Elsegood's site, rich with links to other sites, as well as its own forum and some wonderful newsletters.

e. http://www.LDNscience.org/

Website for physicians. Set up by Moshe Rogosnitzky, this site is important because patients will be able to send their doctors here for more scholarly information about LDN. It contains more detailed information about Dr. Zagon's important research than this book contains.

2. Online LDN Forums

Online forums are places where patients support each other in their use of LDN. Some are Yahoo forums; others are not. Some of these forums concentrate on the use of LDN for specific diseases, such as MS, Parkinson's and cancer; others are more general. See links to forums at http://www.ldners.org/resources.htm#Forums.

3. LDN Studies

a. For a listing of the studies, see *The Faces of Low Dose Naltrexone*: pp 44-52:

http://honestmedicine.typepad.com/ebook-Jan%207%2010--The%20Faces%20of%20Low%20Dose%20Naltrexone.pdf

b. See also http://www.ldners.org/research.htm

c. Here are just a few of the studies that have been conducted on LDN, with very promising results:

i. MS patient/LDN advocate Vicki Finlayson organized a fundraising event. The amount of money raised was enough to fund a small trial at the University of California at San Francisco (UCSF). http://clinicaltrials.gov/ct/show/NCT00501696?order=29 The study has been published in the February 19, 2010 issue of the *Annals of Neurology*, "Pilot trial of Low Dose Naltrexone and quality of life in MS." http://www3.interscience.wiley.com/journal/123289912/abstract

ii. In 2007, a paper describing the results of one study performed at Penn State, titled "Low-dose naltrexone therapy improves active Crohn's disease," *American Journal of Gastroenterology*, 2007 Apr;102(4):820-8. Epub 2007 Jan 11. Smith JP, Stock H, Bingaman S, Mauger D,

Rogosnitzky M, Zagon IS. Department of Medicine, Pennsylvania State University College of Medicine, Hershey, Pennsylvania 17033, USA. http://www.ncbi. nlm.nih.gov/pubmed/17222320

iii. A pilot trial of low-dose naltrexone in primary progressive multiple sclerosis: *Mult Scler.* 2008 Sep;14(8):1076-83. Gironi M, Martinelli-Boneschi F, Sacerdote P, Solaro C, Zaffaroni M, Cavarretta R, Moiola L, Bucello S, Radaelli M, Pilato V, Rodegher M, Cursi M, Franchi S, Martinelli V, Nemni R, Comi G, Martino G. Institute of Experimental Neurology (INSPE) and Department of Neurology, San Raffaele Scientific Institute, Via Olgettina 58, Milan, Italy.

http://www.ncbi.nlm.nih.gov/pubmed/18728058?ordinal pos=5&itool=EntrezSystem2.PEntrez.Pubmed.Pubmed_ ResultsPanel.Pubmed_DefaultReportPanel.Pubmed_RV-DocSu

d. For a more complete listing of LDN trials, please go to Dr. Gluck's website: www.lowdosenaltrexone.org, and SammyJo Wilkinson's website: www.LDNers.org.

4. Compounding Pharmacies Known to Compound LDN Correctly

a. http://www.ldners.org/resources.htm

b. http://www.lowdosenaltrexone.org/comp_pharm.htm

c. http://www.LDNaware.org/: Lists pharmacies by country.

5. Doctors who Prescribe LDN

Go to http://www.lowdosenaltrexone.org, and access the audios and videos of physicians who publicly champion LDN. Among them: Dr. Tom Gilhooly, Dr. Phil Boyle, Dr. Burt Berkson, Dr. David Gluck and others.

6. Dr. Ian Zagon: Primary LDN Researcher

Ian Zagon, PhD is recognized as the researcher who is the LDN champion in the lab. He has done research on LDN, starting in the 1980s, around the same time Dr. Bihari was treating patients with LDN. You may learn more about Dr. Zagon at http://fred.psu.edu/ds/retrieve/fred/investigator/isz1 and http://www.ldnscience.org/low-dose-naltrexone-ldn/ldn-researchers/119.

I would like to explain here that, while I consider Dr. Zagon's research to be important, I feel strongly that, without Dr. Bihari, LDN would never have reached the community of people with autoimmune diseases who need it. After all, Dr. Zagon is a researcher whose work is mostly animal-based. Dr. Bihari treated actual people with actual diseases. My book is about how treatments help actual people—not lab animals.

7. **Media Coverage of Dr. Bihari**

    a. A video of Dr. Bihari with Dr. Pat Crowley, from the 2006 LDN conference. At the bottom of the screen, you'll see several thumbnails. If you scroll to the right, you'll see that Dr. Bihari himself appears several times, interspersed between patient testimonies. I love listening to him talk; he's fascinating.

    http://video.google.com/videoplay?docid=831309287569609 6715&hl=en#

    b. Public radio interview with Dr. Bihari

    In this interview from 2003, Dr. Kamau B. Kokayi talks with Dr. Bihari. I love this interview because of the way Dr. Bihari explains his paradigm-shifting theories. His brilliance and kindness shine through.

    http://www.lowdosenaltrexone.org/gazorpa/interview.html

8. **Dr. Bihari's 2004 proposal to the Irish government to do a trial on LDN for MS, unedited (Courtesy of Mary Boyle Bradley)**

    http://honestmedicine.typepad.com/LDNMSTrial1.pdf

Full Text, unedited and original:

    Multiple Sclerosis Letter of Inquiry Submission
    Contact Information
    Organization Name: The Foundation of Immunological Research

Organization Address:
29 West 15th Street
New York, New York, 10011 USA
Organization Tax Status: 501(c)(3) public charity
Primary Contact Prefix: Dr. Bernard Bihari, MD
Title of Primary Contact: Medical Director
Primary Contact Phone: 001 212 9294196
Primary Contact Email: mboylebradley@msn.com
Primary Contact Fax: 001 212 2299371

Narrative

Naltrexone at doses of 1.75 mg to 4.5 mg has been shown to stabilize the CD4 absolute count and the CD4 percentage in people with HIV/ AIDS. It has also been shown to provide protection from HIV disease, protection as reflected in the incidence of opportunistic infections and HIV related deaths. In the wake of these results Dr. Bihari discovered serendipitously that Low Dose Naltrexone (LDN) because of its ability to increase production of endorphins during the night, when it is taken at bedtime (9 p.m. to 2 a.m.) to be useful in the treatment of a wide range of autoimmune diseases. These diseases apparently respond because of the role low serum endorphins and intracellular endorphins play in their etiology, with return of normal endorphin levels having a beneficial effect.

The autoimmune disease in which LDN is used most at present is Multiple sclerosis (MS). Dr. Bihari currently has 384 patients with MS in his medical care in a private practice setting in New York City. These patients have been on LDN for an average of 2.5 years with a range of 1 week to 19 years. The overall results of treatment with this drug have been excellent. Only 3 of the 384 patients have shown any attacks. To be more specific, one of these three, who started LDN 18 years ago, at the age of 22 in 1988, had one attack after 5 years on the drug, 30 days after stopping it. The patient resumed LDN when the attack appeared and has had none in the 13 years since. The second of the three, a 41 year old woman had an episode of optic neuritis which cleared in 4 weeks, after 18 months on LDN. The last of the three was a patient who experienced an episode of numbness in the left leg after 8 months on LDN, not previously present, which cleared after 3 weeks. The other 381 patients with MS have had no sign of disease activity since starting LDN.

Approximately 25% of the patients starting on 4.5 mg LDN have experienced an increase in spasticity. When the dose is reduced to 3 mg the increase always clears. Overall, most patients with significant spasticity, especially in the legs, experience an overall reduction in spasticity once the proper dose is achieved. The fatigue associated with MS is generally reduced, sometimes substantially after a few days on LDN. Rarely other MS symptoms are reduced while on LDN, such as bladder spasticity and urinary incontinence and there is an occasional patient who shows cognitive improvement if cognitive impairment was present before treatment began.

About 20 percent of these patients were on Avonex, Betaseron, Copaxone, Novantrone or methotrexate before beginning LDN. Although no recommendation is made about whether or not to continue these drugs by Dr. Bihari, only one has remained on Copaxone with LDN for the 12 months she has been on LDN. The Copaxone did not seem to interfere with her LDN effect.

There are at present several thousand people with MS on LDN, who have had their LDN prescribed by their physicians after reading about it on the LDN website, www.LDNinfo.org. Emails to the website as well as emails to a number of other websites devoted to MS treatment suggests that the response to LDN in the wider community of people with MS approximates the clinical response in Dr. Bihari's medical practice.

Background

In the light of recent evidence suggesting that the endorphinergic system plays an important role in the homeostatic regulation of immune function, we have developed and tested immunoenhancing treatment using Low Dose Naltrexone in the dosage range of 1.75 to 4.5 mg. Human T-cell rosette formation is enhanced by metenkephalin and this effect is blocked by prior or simultaneous treatment with naltrexone, a narcotic antagonist, thus demonstrating that T-cells have functionally important opiate receptors. Other studies have shown that the following functions involve opiate receptors and/or are facilitated by endorphins: lymphocyte blastogenesis, T and B cell cooperation, lymphocyte mitogen responsiveness, in vitro antibody response to sheep RBC-c, natural killer cell activity, expression of cell surface markers involved in lymphocyte activation (such as OKT10,IL2, and la receptors), monocyte chemotaxis, and macrophage cytotoxicity. Studies indicating that virus infected lymphocytes produce beta-endorphin, and that both Interleukin I and Interleukin II stimulate pituitary synthesis of beta-endorphin, suggest that the central nervous system and the immune system have complex endorphinergic feedback loops that may be important in homeostatic regulation of immune function.

Endorphinergic system involvement in homeostatic regulation of immune function raises the possibility that disturbances in this system may contribute to the pathophysiology of autoimmune diseases such as multiple sclerosis and that endorphinergic upregulation might have an immunoenhancing effect in its treatment.

Project Objective

To demonstrate LDN (low dose naltrexone) as the most effective treatment for Multiple Sclerosis.

Project Description

The first goal of the project is to interest a country in conducting a full-scale, double-blind, placebo-controlled prospective study of LDN as a treatment for MS. Then, with the successful outcome of the clinical trial, Dr. Bihari will work to achieve these further objectives:

1. In the country which hosted the trial, to license a capable entity—with no licensing fee—to manufacture LDN.
2. To help ensure the general availability of LDN throughout the world.
3. To gain scientific recognition of the efficacy of LDN for the treatment of MS.

Trial Proposal

A 12-month placebo controlled study of LDN at 3 mg is planned. Recommended sample size is 300 patients, 2/3 on the drug, 1/3 on placebo. Patients should be randomly assigned to drug or placebo. If the trial shows efficacy the placebo patients should be offered LDN when the trial is completed.

Patient Eligibility

Patients must be between 18 and 65 years of age with relapsing, remitting or secondary progressive MS. Patients with primary progressive MS may not participate.

Study Design

Patients will have initial medical and neurological history and physical exams with review of medical records to determine if they are eligible. All patients considered eligible should have had at least one MRI of the brain, the spinal cord or both showing plaques/demyelination consistent with a diagnosis of MS. On the trial entry patients will be randomly assigned to active drug or placebo. Patients on drug will be started at 3 mg of LDN taken between 9 p.m. and 2 a.m. Within one week of admission to the study all patients should receive an MRI of the brain and the spinal cord to be repeated at the end of the study.

Study Evaluations

Patients will undergo a complete medical/neurological and physical exam every 8 weeks for 12 months.

Monitoring Procedure

Case Report forms will be developed for entering data on admission and on the 8 week visits. Presumably the patients will be seen on these visits by a physician, physician's assistant or nurse practitioner. An independent monitoring agency should collect data from the Case Report Forms for analysis at the end of the trial.

Side Effects
Naltrexone has some mild side effects at 50 mg per day. In several thousand patients taking it at a low dose, most recently 3 to 4.5 mg, no side effects or adverse reactions have been observed except for 1-2% of patients who experience restless sleep at this dose for brief period.

Pregnancy
No teratogenic effects have been observed with naltrexone at 50 mg or at the lower doses of 1.75 to 4.5 mg. However, there is a theoretical possibility that raising endorphins, which are always low in people with autoimmune diseases, might reduce birth weights of babies born to mothers on the drug by as much as 10 percent. Because of this, a pregnancy test should be done routinely in women of childbearing age applying for admission to the study and if it is positive they should be excluded, as should women who get pregnant during the course of the study. This problem is probably minor and ultimately may not affect the usefulness of the drug in pregnant women because of the seriousness of the illness it is being used to treat. However, pregnant women should be excluded from this trial until more information is available about the effects of LDN on pregnancy.

Informed Consent
The investigator is responsible to ensure that each subject (or subject's legal representative) signs an informed consent statement prior to participation in this trial. The consent form and the whole protocol should be reviewed and approved by an appropriate Institutional Review Board to assure protection of patient's rights. The signed copies of the consent forms are to be retained by the investigator. The patient will be informed of his or her right to privacy and the fact that the results will be submitted only to the study sponsor and the appropriate department of the hospital in such a way that the patient's identity will not be known. The Institutional Review Board and the hospital have the right to inspect the patient's medical record to verify the accuracy and completeness of this trial.

Amount Requested to Complete LDN for MS Trial in Ireland
900,000 Euros

Project Duration
12 months

9. **LDN Fact Sheets to Educate Your Doctor About LDN**

   a. Patient Guide: How to Talk to Your Doctor About LDN:
   http://www.lowdosenaltrexone.org/gazorpa/PatientGuide.html

   b. To My Doctor:
   http://www.ldnaware.org/uploadeddocuments/to-my-doctor.pdf

   c. Low Dose Naltrexone Fact Sheet:
   http://www.ldnresearchtrustfiles.co.uk/docs/LDN%20English%20Fact%20Sheet.pdf

10. Honest Medicine's Articles About LDN

I have written several articles about LDN. They are all contained here:
http://www.honestmedicine.com/low-dose-naltrexone/

REMINDER:

As I pointed out on page 28 of this book, it is extremely challenging to format electronic links in a printed book. Therefore, you may find it difficult to use the links as published in *Honest Medicine*. If you do, please go to http://www.HonestMedicine.com/hyperlinks.html for a complete list of the links in this book. They were all correct at the time of publication.

About the Author

Julia Schopick was perfectly poised to write *Honest Medicine*. She credits her parents for giving her the courage to follow her own gut and tell the truth as she sees it about the state of medical care in the United States. Her maternal grandmother turned down conventional medical care in the late 1920s in favor of then-experimental cancer treatments abroad, and her father was a "rebel doctor" before it became fashionable to be one. From the 1950s until his death in 1976, her dad was highly critical of the medical system and of his fellow doctors, and had some pretty salty things to say about both. Add to this Julia's own experience as a public relations consultant, with several clients in the holistic health field, and you have the "perfect person" to write *Honest Medicine*.

It wasn't until 1990, though, when Julia's late husband Tim Fisher was diagnosed with a very serious brain cancer that she witnessed, up close and personal, the vast array of deficiencies in the medical system. She discovered that doctors didn't necessarily share with their patients—or even know about—the best possible treatments for their unique personal situations. It is these deficiencies that Julia has set out to expose both on her website and in this book, in her role as patient advocate. Her aim is to help others navigate their way through serious healthcare mazes to find the right treatments for them.

To do this, Julia has combined her writing skills and her promotional abilities. She's written several guest columns for professional publications, including *American Medical News*, the AMA publication, on the topic of doctor-patient communications; *ADVANCE*, the professional publication for physical therapists; and *SEARCH*, the National Brain Tumor Foundation newsletter. In addition, she has written guest columns about cutting-edge treatments like those featured in this book for *Alternative and Complementary Therapies*, a publication for holistic health practitioners. Her work and essays on medical topics have also been featured in the *British Medical Journal, Modern Maturity* and the *Chicago Sun-Times.*

Julia's book represents the next step in her career as a patient advocate, teaching an even wider audience about actual treatments their doctors may not know about, and might not tell their patients about, even if they did know about them.

Julia is passionate about spreading the word through speaking engagements, articles in the press and media appearances. Please contact her at Julia@HonestMedicine.com to discuss ways she might educate your group through public presentations or articles for your publication. Julia is also available for media interviews on topics related to the issues covered in this book and on her website, www.HonestMedicine.com.

Index

CPSIA information can be obtained
at www.ICGtesting.com
Printed in the USA
LVOW10s2345030417
529495LV00011B/700/P